Gail Rae-Garwood

When my family doctor told me ten years ago that I probably had a problem and it had to do with my kidneys, maybe Chronic Kidney Disease, my first reaction was to demand in no uncertain terms, "What is it and how did I get it?" Hence, the title of my first CKD book.

There are many, many of us out there. By us, I mean those who have Chronic Kidney Disease. Friends and family of CKD patients can also gain some insight into the daily travails of living with the disease via this book of 2017's *SlowItDownCKD* blogs. This is not an improvement over the last books in the *SlowItDownCKD* series, but an addition which covers topics I hadn't thought of in previous years or those that readers asked about last year.

I am no expert, but I did want to know what was happening to me on a daily basis, what the medications that were ordered for me were supposed to do, and what new discoveries there were that might help slow down this deterioration of my kidneys. Apparently, so do my readers. That's what this collection of 2017's blogs is about.

The more you know about Chronic Kidney Disease, the more comfortable you'll feel in the early or moderate stages of having the disease yourself. I sure wish someone had blogged about it when it was new to me.

I've discovered I have something like 17,000 readers in 106 countries and they're not afraid to tell me what they want to know. I research for them and respond with a blog post, but remind them they need to speak with their nephrologist and/or renal nutritionist before taking any action. And I repeatedly remind my readers that I am not a doctor.

I've written other books about Chronic Kidney Disease that you'll find referenced many times in the blogs. Those books are ***What Is***

It and How Did I Get It? Early Stage Chronic Kidney Disease, The Book of Blogs: Moderate Stage Chronic Kidney Disease, Part 1; The Book of Blogs: Moderate Stage Chronic Kidney Disease, Part 2; SlowItDownCKD 2015, and *SlowItDownCKD 2016.* You'll notice *The Book of Blogs: Moderate Stage Chronic Kidney Disease, Part 1* is not hyperlinked. That's because I replaced this unwieldy book with two books: *SlowItDownCKD 2011* and *SlowItDownCKD 2012.* My plan is to do the same with *The Book of Blogs: Moderate Stage Chronic Kidney Disease, Part 2* later this year.

In the interest of keeping this book from becoming mammoth, I've removed the pictures, diagrams, dead links, and news of past events, although at my readers' request, I've included URLs. I also removed my signature closing: "Until next week, keep living your life!" After all, how many times can you read the same sentence in a single book?

Welcome to *SlowItDownCKD 2017.*

Keep living your life,
Gail

p.s. I want Bear to know how much I STILL appreciate his respecting Monday as blog day, and when I'm writing a book, Monday, Tuesday, Wednesday, Thursday, Friday, Saturday, and Sunday as writing days. You're one of a kind, honey.

1/2/17 *Starting the New Year with a Miracle*
Happy New Year and welcome to 2017. A new year brings to mind new beginnings... and that leads me to Part 3 of the miracle series, as promised. I am so, so serious about this and hope you decide to take on for yourself causing a miracle in CKD by sharing information.

I was thinking about social media the other day. Where are the public service announcements about Chronic Kidney Disease? I am still – nine years after my diagnosis – knocking on seemingly closed doors to encourage Public Service Announcements everywhere. While the public doesn't seem as involved with network television or radio as they were when I was younger, we now have Twitter, Facebook, Instagram, LinkedIn, and Tumblr to name just a few ways we can share.

I use a both a *Facebook* page and a *Twitter* account to post one fact about or information pertinent to those with CKD daily. Join me at *SlowItDownCKD* on Facebook and *@SlowItDownCKD* on Twitter. You may not want to do this, but feel free to 'steal' the information posted and share it with others.

There are also Podcasts, Internet Radio Shows, YouTubes, etc. to share what the public needs to know about CKD. A *YouTube* can be viewed by one person who posts it on *Facebook* and go viral. Don't bother looking at mine. They're pretty painful. I'll look into this again at a later date.

On the other hand, these are some of the social media venues that interviewed me: *The Edge Podcast* 5/9/16, *Online with Andrea* 3/23/15 & 3/07/12, *What Is It? How Did I Get It?* 2/17/12, and *Improve Your Kidney Health with Dr. Rich Snyder, DO* 11/21/11. I never knew these venues existed before I started working towards the miracle I wanted to cause.

Lo and behold, my sharing brought others who wanted to know about CKD, so I was profiled by *Nutrition Action Healthletter, Center for Science in the Public Interest* 9/16, *New York State United Teachers* 'It's What We Do' 8/9/16, and *Wall Street Journal* 'Health Matters' 1/13/14.

Let's say you agree that sharing can cause a miracle in Chronic Kidney Disease and want to join in living a life causing this miracle. The first thing you'd want to do is learn about CKD. The American Kidney Fund and the National Kidney Foundation both have a wealth of information written for the lay person, not the medical community. By the way, the National Kidney Foundation also has information about CKD globally. Maybe you'd rather join in World Kidney Day gatherings and distribute materials. Then keep an eye on World Kidney Day's *Twitter* account for locations around the world.

As you can see, I've been creating this miracle is by writing for these organizations and more kidney specific ones, as well as guest blogging for various groups. You may not choose to do that... but you can speak at your religious group meetings, your sports league, your weekly card game, or whatever other group you're comfortable with.

A miracle doesn't have to be profound. You can help create this one. All you need is a little education about CKD and the willingness to introduce the subject where you haven't before.

I live my life expecting miracles and I find they happen. This miracle that I'm causing – and is happening – has been (and is) created by sharing, sharing, sharing. The more than 200 million people who have Chronic Kidney Disease need this information, to say nothing of those who have yet to be diagnosed.

There aren't that many organs to go around for those who didn't know they had CKD and progressed to End Stage Renal Disease. We know that transplantation is a treatment, not a cure, and one that doesn't always last forever. We also know that kidneys from living donors usually last longer than those from cadaver donors. Share that, too.

We have our no cost, no pain, no tools needed miracle right on our lips... or at our fingertips. Start sharing, keep sharing, urge others to share, and help to prevent or slow down the progression in the decline of kidneys worldwide. Sharing is causing a miracle in CKD. Both deaths and hospitalizations for this disease have declined since 2008. If that isn't a miracle, I don't know what is. I keep saying I live my life expecting miracles; this is one of them.

I was a private person before this disease. Now, in addition to the Facebook page and Twitter accounts, I make use of an Instagram account (*SlowItDownCKD*) where I post an eye catching picture daily with the hash tag *#SlowItDownCKD*. This brings people to my weekly blog about CKD and the four books I wrote about it: one explaining it and the others the blogs in print – rather than electronic form for those who don't have a computer or are not computer savvy. Time consuming? Oh yes, but if I expect to live a life of miracles, I need to contribute that time to share what I can about the disease and urge others to do the same.

I am urging you to realize you are the others I am asking to help cause a miracle in Chronic Kidney Disease. As the Rabbinic sage Hillel the Elder said, "If I am not for myself, who will be for me? If I am only for myself, what am I? If not now, when?" Now. You. Me. Others. CKD.

1/9/17 *Where Does It All Come From?*
For the past two weeks, I've had the flu. I've missed the Chanukah Gathering at my own house, Kwanzaa, and New Year's. I even missed my neighbor's husband/son birthday party and a seminar I enjoy attending.

Before you ask, yes I did have a flu shot. However, Strain A seems to be somewhat resistant to that. True, I have been able to cut down on the severity of the flu by taking the shot, but it leaves me with a burning question: How can anyone produce as much mucus as I have in the last two weeks?

Mucus. Snot. Sputum. Secretion. Phlegm. Whatever you call it, what is it and how is it produced? According to The Medical Dictionary at http://medical-dictionary.thefreedictionary.com/mucus, it's "the free slime of the mucous membranes, composed of secretion of the glands, various salts, desquamated cells, and leukocytes." By the way, spelling it mucous makes it an adjective, a word that describes a noun. Mucus is the noun, the thing itself. Let's go back to that definition for a minute. We know from *What Is It and How Did I Get It? Early Stage Chronic Kidney Disease* that "Leukocytes are one of the white blood cells that fight bacterial infection." Interesting, the flu as bacterial infection.

Yep, I looked it up and found this on WebMd at http://www.webmd.com/cold-and-flu/tc/flu-signs-of-bacterial-infection-topic-overview: "A bacterial infection may develop following infection with viral influenza." Oh, so that's what all the mucus is about. There's quite a bit more information on this site, but I'm having a hard enough time sticking to my topic as it is. I still wanted to know how mucus (without the 'o') was produced.

Many thanks to Virtual Medical Centre at http://www.myvmc.com/medical-centres/lungs-breathing/anatomy-and-physiology-of-the-nasal-cavity-inner-nose-and-mucosa/ for their help in explaining the following: The nasal cavity refers to the interior of the nose, or the structure which opens exteriorly at the nostrils. It is the entry point for inspired air and the first of a series of structures which form the respiratory system. The cavity is entirely lined by the nasal mucosa, one of the anatomical structures (others include skin, body encasements like the skull and non-nasal mucosa such as those of the vagina and bowel) which form the physical barriers of the body's immune system. These barriers provide mechanical protection from the invasion of infectious and allergenic pathogens.

By now you're probably questioning what this has to do with Chronic Kidney Disease. I found this on a site with the unlikely name Straightdope at http://www.straightdope.com/columns/read/1246/how-does-my-nose-produce-so-much-snot-so-fast-when-i-have-a-cold : "The reason you have a seemingly inexhaustible supply of mucus when suffering from a cold is that the mucus-producing cells lining your nasal cavity extract the stuff mostly from your blood, of which needless to say you have a vast supply. The blood transports the raw materials (largely water) from other parts of the body. Fluid from your blood diffuses through the capillary walls and into the cells and moments later winds up in your handkerchief. (This process isn't unique to mucus; blood is the highway for most of your bodily fluids.)"

While this is not the most scholarly site I've quoted, it offers a simple explanation. Blood. Think about that. I turned to *The Book of Blogs: Moderate Stage Chronic Kidney Disease, Part 1* for help with my explanation.

"Our kidneys are very busy organs, indeed. They produce urine, remove potentially harmful waste products from the blood, aid in the maintenance of the local environment around the cells of the body, help to stimulate the production of red blood cells, regulate blood pressure, help regulate various substances in the blood {For example, potassium, sodium, calcium and more}, help to regulate the acidity of the blood, and regulate the amount of water in the body. Mind you, these are just their main jobs. I haven't even mentioned their minor ones."

Get it? Kidneys filter the blood. Our kidneys are not doing such a great job of filtering our blood since we have CKD, which means we also have compromised immune systems. Thank you for that little gift, CKD. (She wrote sarcastically.)

Now you have the flu. Now what? Here are some hints taken from Dr. Leslie Spry's 'Flu Season and Your Kidneys' reprinted in *The Book of Blogs: Moderate Stage Chronic Kidney Disease, Part 2.* Dr. Spry is an active member of the Public Policy Committee at the National Kidney Foundation, and, I am honored to say, a follower on Twitter.

You should get plenty of rest and avoid other individuals who are ill, in order to limit the spread of the disease. If you are ill, stay home and rest. You should drink plenty of fluids ...to stay well hydrated. You should eat a balanced diet. If you have gastrointestinal illness including nausea, vomiting or diarrhea, you should contact your physician. Immodium® is generally safe to take to control diarrhea. If you become constipated, medications that contain polyethylene glycol, such as Miralax® and Glycolax® are safe to take. You should avoid laxatives that contain magnesium and phosphates. Gastrointestinal illness can lead to dehydration or may keep you from taking your proper medication. If you are on a diuretic, it may not be a good idea to keep taking that diuretic if you are unable to keep liquids down or if you are experiencing diarrhea. You should monitor your temperature and blood pressure carefully and report concerns to your physician. Any medication you take should be reported to your physician...

Check the National Kidney Foundation itself for even more advice in addition to some suggestions as to how to avoid the flu in the first place.

Every year I decide not to write about the flu again. Every year I do. I think I'm oh-so-careful about my health, yet I end up with the flu every year. Sometimes I wonder if these blogs are for you...or reminders for me. Either way, I'm hoping you're able to avoid the flu and keep yourself healthy. That would be another kind of miracle, wouldn't it?

1/16/17 *What Are You Doing for Others?*

Today is Martin Luther King's birthday. Today, more than ever, we need to heed his message. Whether you apply it to today's bizarre political scene, your local community, your family, your co-workers doesn't matter. What matters is the operant word: doing. These words got me to thinking. What AM I doing for others? And what still needs to be done?

My commitment is to spread awareness of Chronic Kidney Disease (CKD). As a patient myself, I know how important this is. As you know, CKD is a costly, lethal disease if not caught early and treated… and it's not just older folks – like me – who are at risk. One out of ten people worldwide has CKD, yet an overwhelming number of them are unaware they have it.

We also know the disease can be treated, just not the way you'd usually expect a disease to be treated. A diet with restrictions on protein, potassium, phosphorous and sodium is one aspect of that treatment. Exercise, adequate sleep, and avoiding stress are some of the other aspects. Some patients – like me – may have to take medication for their high blood pressure since that also affects kidney function. Imagine preventing a death with lifestyle changes. Now image saving the lives of all those who don't know they have CKD by making them aware this disease exists. Powerful, isn't it?

We're all aware by now that the basic method of diagnosing CKD is via routine blood and urine tests. Yet, many people do not undergo these tests during doctor or clinic visits, so don't know they have Chronic Kidney Disease, much less start treating it. That's where I come in; I tell people what can be done. I tell people how they can be diagnosed and treated, if necessary.

I was a private person before this CKD diagnosis so many years ago. Now, in addition to a Facebook page, LinkedIn, and Twitter accounts as *SlowItDownCKD*, I make use of an Instagram account where I post an eye catching picture daily with the hashtag *#SlowItDownCKD*. This brings people to my weekly blog about CKD (the one you're reading now) and the five books I wrote about it: *What Is It and How Did I Get It? Early Stage Chronic Kidney Disease* (which explains CKD) and the others – *The Book of Blogs: Moderate Stage Chronic Kidney Disease, Part 1; The Book of Blogs: Moderate Stage Chronic Kidney Disease, Part 2; SlowItDownCKD 2015 and SlowItDownCKD 2016* – which are the blogs in print for those who don't have a computer or are not computer savvy. *The Book of Blogs: Moderate Stage Chronic Kidney Disease, Part 1* has since been separated into *SlowItCKD 2011* and *SlowItDownCKD 2012* since it was so unwieldy. My plan is to do the same for *The Book of Blogs: Moderate Stage Chronic Kidney Disease, Part 2*

Healthline at https://www.healthline.com/ is a well-respected, informative site for medical information. This past year this blog, *SlowItDownCKD*, was a winner in their list of The Six Best Kidney Disease Blogs. That brought the hits on my page up by the hundreds. That means hundreds more people are now aware of Chronic Kidney Disease, how it is diagnosed, how it is treated, and how to live with it.

But not everything is working as I'd hoped it would. Unfortunately, I am still not having success in having Public Service Announcements placed on television or radio. Nor have I been able to interest most general magazines or newspapers in bringing the disease to the public's awareness.

It hasn't totally been a wipeout there, though. Michael Garcia did interview me on **The Edge Podcast** and both **Nutrition Action Healthletter, Center for Science in the Public Interest** (the nation's largest-circulation nutrition newsletter) and **New York State United Teachers** (membership 600,000) **'It's What We Do'** profiled my work spreading CKD Awareness. Profiling my work, interviewing me, mentioning the blog all bring awareness of Chronic Kidney Disease to the public. Awareness leads to testing. Testing leads to diagnosing. Diagnosing leads to treatment. Treatment leads to saving lives. This is why I do what I can to spread awareness of Chronic Kidney Disease.

What about you? Can you speak about CKD with your family? Your friends? Your co-workers? Your brothers and sisters in whichever religion you follow? What about your neighbors? I was surprised and delighted at the number of non CKD friends and neighbors who follow the blog. When I asked why they did, they responded, "I have a friend…." We may all have a friend who may have CKD, whether that friend has told us yet or not.

There are more formal methods of spreading this awareness if that interests you. The National Kidney Foundation has an Advocacy Network.

"A NKF Advocate is someone who has been affected by kidney disease, donation or transplant and who wants to empower and educate others. These include people with kidney disease, dialysis patients, transplant recipients, living donors, donor family members, caregivers, friends and family members.

Advocacy plays an integral role in our mission. You can make a significant difference in the lives of kidney patients by representing the National Kidney Foundation. We give you the tools you need to make your voice heard."

You can read more about this program at https://www.kidney.org/node/17759 or you can call 1.800.622.9010 for more information.

The American Kidney Fund also has an advocacy program, but it's a bit different.

"There is strength in numbers. More than 5,100 passionate patients, friends, loved ones and kidney care professionals in our Advocacy Network are making a huge difference on Capitol Hill and in their own communities. Together, we are fighting for policies that improve care for patients, protect patients' access to health insurance and increase funding for kidney research. As advocates, we play a key role in educating elected officials and our communities about the impact of kidney disease."

You can register for this network online at http://www.kidneyfund.org/advocacy/advocate-for-kidney-patients/advocacy-network/

Obviously, I'm serious about **doing** that which will spread awareness of CKD. You can take a gander at my website, gail-raegarwood.com, to see if that sparks any ideas for you as to how you can start doing something about spreading awareness of CKD, too. I urge you to do whatever you can, wherever you can, and whenever you can.

1/23/17 *It's Unfolding Now*
Remember when I was lucky enough to catch the flu just after Christmas? (She wrote sarcastically.) When I went to the Immediate Care facility my doctor is associated with, the doctor there had my records and knew I'd had pleurisy at one time. But now, he ordered a chest x-ray to check for pneumonia. What he found instead was news to me... so, of course, I'm telling you about it.

To quote from the final result report of the X-ray: "There is unfolding of the thoracic aorta." Huh? In **The Book of Blogs: Moderate Stage Chronic Kidney Disease, Part 1** there's an explanation of thorax.

"What? The what? Oh, the thorax. That's 'the part of the human body between the neck and the diaphragm, partially encased by the ribs and containing the heart and lungs; the chest' according to The Free Dictionary at http://www.thefreedictionary.com/thorax."

Thoracic is the adjective form of thorax; it describes the aorta in this case.

Do you remember what the aorta is? I sort of, kind of did, but figured I'd better make certain before I started writing about it. MedicineNet at http://www.medicinenet.com/script/main/art.asp?articlekey=229 5 was helpful here.

"The aorta gives off branches that go to the head and neck, the arms, the major organs in the chest and abdomen, and the legs. It serves to supply them all with oxygenated blood. The aorta is the central conduit from the heart to the body."

Now I get the connection between Chronic Kidney Disease and the aorta. Did you catch "oxygenated blood" in that definition?

And what organs oxygenate the blood? Right. Your kidneys. This excerpt from *SlowItDownCKD 2015* may help.

""The National Kidney and Urologic Diseases Information Clearinghouse ...explains.

'Healthy kidneys produce a hormone called erythropoietin, or EPO, which stimulates the bone marrow to produce the proper number of red blood cells needed to carry oxygen to vital organs. Diseased kidneys, however, often don't make enough EPO. As a result, the bone marrow makes fewer red blood cells.'"

With me so far? Now, what the heck is an unfolded aorta? I turned to the British site for radiologists, Radiopaedia.org, at https://radiopaedia.org/articles/unfolded-aorta for the definition. "The term **unfolded aorta** refers to the widened and 'opened up' appearance of the aortic arch on a frontal chest radiograph. It is one of the more common causes for apparent mediastinal widening and is seen with increasing age.

It occurs due to the discrepancy in the growth of the ascending aorta with age, where the length of the ascending aorta increases out of proportion with diameter, causing the plane of the arch to swivel."

I purposely left the click through definitions in so you read them for yourself. You know the drill: click on the link while holding down your control key. For those of you who are reading the print version of the blog, just add the definition of aorta to the common terms we know: arch and ascending.

Mediastinal, according to the Merriam-Webster Dictionary at https://www.merriam-webster.com/dictionary/mediastinum is the adjective (describing) form of mediastinum or "the space in the chest between the pleural sacs of the lungs that contains all the tissues and organs of the chest except the lungs and pleurae; *also*: this space with its contents."

Hang on there, folks, just one more definition. I searched for a new site that wouldn't offer a terribly technical definition of pleura (or pleurae) and found this at verywell.com.

"The pleura refers to the 2 membranes that cover the lungs and line the chest cavity. The purpose of the pleura is to cushion the lungs during respiration.

The pleural cavity is the space between these 2 membranes and contains pleural fluid."

Side note: I definitely feel like I'm back teaching a college class again.

Okay, so now we have a bunch of definitions, we've put them together as best we can and where does it bring us? Are you ready for this? Nowhere. An unfolding of the thoracic aorta is nothing more than a function of age.

However, with CKD, it's somewhere. As was explained in **What Is It and How Did I Get It? Early Stage Chronic Kidney Disease,** "**Hemoglobin** is the protein in red blood cells that carries oxygen from the lungs to the rest of the body." We're already not getting enough oxygen due to our poor, declining in function kidneys.

Am I concerned about the unfolding thoracic aorta? No, not at all. It happens with age; I don't think I can do anything about that. But, the CKD that also lowers our oxygen production? Oh yes, I can – do – and will do something about that by protecting my kidneys as best I can and keeping the remaining kidney function I have.

Kidneys.com, quoted in *The Book of Blogs: Moderate Stage Chronic Kidney Disease, Part 1,* did a nice job of laying out a plan for me to do just that.

"Along with taking your prescribed blood pressure medications, lifestyle changes such as losing weight, exercising, meditating, eating less sodium, drinking less alcohol and quitting smoking can help lower blood pressure. Better blood pressure control helps preserve kidney function."

I added using my sleep apnea machine and aiming for eight hours of sleep a night. I also stick to my renal diet – which limits protein, phosphorous, potassium, and sodium (as mentioned by kidney.com) – for the most part and keeping my kidneys hydrated by drinking at least 64 ounces of fluid a day.

Is it hard? I don't know any more. It's been nine years. They're simply habits I've developed to live as long as I can and, sometimes, even raise the function of my kidneys.

When my New York daughter was with us over the holidays, I realized how differently we eat than other people do. My husband has chosen to pretty much eat the way I do. So she actually had to go down to the market to pick up the foods that people ordinarily eat. It would have been funny if I hadn't been sick. I would have gone with her and laughed each time I answered, "No," when she asked, "Do you eat this?"

2/6/17 *The Three Musketeers*

I was in Cuba last week with very sketchy internet, so it was not possible to post a blog. But for now, I was thinking about a friend – you know, one of those Facebook friends you never met but you feel an instant kinship with – who told me that her surgeon warned her that her recovery from the spinal fusion surgery she'd recently had would be slow because she has Chronic Kidney Disease.

CKD...bone healing. Let's start slowly and work this one out. First of all, what do the kidneys have to do with your bones?

I turned to **What Is It and How Did I Get It? Early Stage Chronic Kidney Disease** for some answers.

"Both vitamin D and calcium are needed for strong bones. It is yet another job of your kidneys to keep your bones strong and healthy....Vitamin D enables the calcium from the food you eat to be absorbed in the body. CKD may leech the calcium from your bones and body....Be aware that kidney disease can cause excessive phosphorus. And what does that mean for Early Stage CKD patients? Not much if the phosphorous levels are kept low. Later, at Stages 4 and 5, bone problems including pain and breakage may be endured since excess phosphorous means the body tries to maintain balance by using the calcium that should be going to the bones."

Whoa! Each one of those thoughts needs at least a bit more explanation. Let's start with the jobs of the kidneys. *The Book of Blogs: Moderate Stage Chronic Kidney Disease, Part 1* has a paragraph that mentions some of them. I turned it into a list to make it more visual.

"Our kidneys are very busy organs, indeed. They produce urine, remove potentially harmful waste products from the blood, aid in the maintenance of the local environment around the cells of the body, help to stimulate the production of red blood cells, regulate blood pressure, help regulate various substances in the blood {For example, potassium, sodium, calcium and more}, help to regulate the acidity of the blood, and regulate the amount of water in the body. Mind you, these are just their main jobs."

Another of those various substances in the blood they help to regulate is phosphorous. That's where one of the connections between CKD and your bones lies. If your phosphorous is not being correctly regulated by your kidneys (since your kidneys are impaired), yes you do experience pain and broken bones, but did you notice that your body also diverts your necessary-for-bone-health calcium to regulate the other substances in your blood?

I wanted to know more about phosphorous so I turned to *The Book of Blogs: Moderate Stage Chronic Kidney Disease, Part 2*. I got a chuckle from seeing that I'd quoted from my first book in explaining how phosphorous works. I'd forgotten about that.

"This is the second most plentiful mineral in the body and works closely with the first, calcium. Together, they produce strong bones and teeth. 85% of the phosphorous and calcium in our bodies is stored in the bones and teeth. The rest circulates in the blood except for about 5% that is in cells and tissues…. Phosphorous balances and metabolizes other vitamins and minerals including vitamin D which is so important to CKD patients. As usual, it performs other functions, such as getting oxygen to tissues and changing protein, fat and carbohydrate into energy."

Talk about multi-tasking. Let's focus in on the calcium/phosphorous connection. Kidney Health Australia explained this succinctly:

"When your kidney function declines, you are unable to get rid of excess phosphate. (Me here: that's what we call phosphorous except when dealing with inorganic chemistry.) The phosphate builds up in your body and binds to calcium, which, in turn, lowers your calcium levels. When your calcium levels get too low, glands in your neck (called the parathyroid glands) pull the extra calcium your body needs out of your bones. This can make your bones easy to break. The bound phosphate and calcium get deposited in your blood vessels. It can increase your risk of heart disease and stroke. It can also cause skin ulcers and lumps in your joints."

So where does vitamin D come in? As was mentioned in **SlowItDownCKD 2015,**

"'Vitamin D: Regulates calcium and phosphorous blood levels as well as promoting bone formation, among other tasks – affects the immune system.' We know vitamin D can be a real problem for us. How many of you are taking vitamin D supplements? Notice my hand is raised, too. How many of you read the blogs about vitamin D? Good!"

It sounds like vitamin D is in charge here. Let me get some more information about that for us. Bingo: DaVita at https://www.davita.com/kidney-disease/diet-and-nutrition/diet-basics/vitamin-d-and-chronic-kidney-disease/e/5326 was able to help us out here.

"Vitamin D is responsible for:
- Building and maintaining strong bones
- Keeping the right level of calcium and phosphorus in the blood
- Preventing bones from becoming weak or malformed
- Preventing rickets in children and osteomalacia in adults
- too much vitamin D can be toxic…."

Hmmm, the three work together with vitamin D as their captain. I wondered what foods would be helpful for my friend in her healing process.

"Calcium
Milk, yogurt, cheese, sardines, spinach, collard greens, kale, soybeans, black-eyed peas, white beans and foods often fortified with calcium: breakfast cereals, orange juice, soy milk, rice milk

Vitamin D
Salmon, mackerel, sardines, tuna, flounder, sole, cod
Phosphorus
Ricotta cheese, barley, soybeans, sunflower seeds, cottage cheese, lentils"

Thank you to Weill Cornell Medical College's Women's Health Advisor for the above information.

But, you know, it's never just that easy. As CKD patients, we have limits of how much protein, potassium, sodium, and – wait for it – phosphorous we can eat each day. There is no socking in all the good stuff for kidney disease patients.

I can see why my friend's surgeon told her the recovery might be slow. Something else that keeps the bones strong is weight bearing exercise, but how can she do that right now?

2/13/17 *I'm Wearing Out*

I'll hold off the Cuba blog for another week because something else seems more relevant right now. I was thinking about last week's blog and what my friend's surgeon told her about slow bone healing when you have Chronic Kidney Disease. Some vague memory was nagging me. And then I got it. Yay for those times we conquer mind fog.

Remember I'd had the flu that morphed into a secondary infection recently? My breathing was so wheezy and I was feeling so poorly that I went back to immediate care a second time just ten days after the first time I'd been there.

What is immediate care you ask? That's a good question. Let's allow HonorHealth at https://www.honorhealth.com/medical-services/immediate-care-urgent-care to answer.

"If you need medical care quickly for a non-life-threating illness or injury.... Patients of all ages can walk into any one of the four HonorHealth Medical Group immediate care centers, with no appointment needed, for such ailments and injuries as lacerations, back pain, cough, headache, or sinus or urinary tract infections.

...advantages:
- Your co-pay is lower with immediate care compared to urgent care.
- All four Valley locations are within offices of HonorHealth primary care physicians. That means any follow-up care you might need will be easy to access.
- Your medical records, including labs and radiology images, soon will be linked systemwide with other HonorHealth facilities. So if you find yourself in an HonorHealth hospital or at an HonorHealth specialist, your medical information will be easily accessible by trusted caregivers. In

addition, you won't need to provide the same information over and over again; it will be in your medical record."

It's also clean, well equipped, and the wait is never too long. That's where I go when I can't get an appointment with my primary care doctor. There may be a different immediate care facility in your area.

Back to the bone issue. While I was there, an x-ray of my chest was ordered to check for pneumonia. I'm lucky: there wasn't any. But, there was the unfolding of the thoracic aorta which I blogged about, and there was "levoconvex curvature and degenerative spurring of the thoracic spine."

I am way past the point of panicking when I encounter a medical term I don't know in a report about my body, but I am still curious… very curious. As I wrote in the blog about the unfolding aorta:

".... In *The Book of Blogs: Moderate Stage Chronic Kidney Disease, Part 1* there's an explanation of thorax. …

'the part of the human body between the neck and the diaphragm, partially encased by the ribs and containing the heart and lungs; the chest'

according to The Free Dictionary
at http://www.thefreedictionary.com/thorax.

Thoracic is the adjective form of thorax."

Adjectives describe the noun – the person, place, thing, or idea.

And degenerative? There's a poignant discovery about that in *What Is It and How Did I Get It? Early Stage Chronic Kidney Disease*:

"Ah, CKD is a degenerative disease."

Well, all right then. Both CKD and the spurring of my thoracic spine are degenerative. What exactly does degenerative mean, though? My all-time favorite Merriam-Webster Dictionary tells us it's the adjective (yep, that means describing) form of degeneration. Their definition of degeneration is

"deterioration of a tissue or an organ in which its function is diminished or its structure is impaired."

This doesn't sound too great; it sounds like CKD.

What about "levoconvex curvature"? I understand curvature and I'm sure you do, too, so let's just deal with levoconvex. I see convex in the word and know that means curving outward. Levo is new to me. GLOBALRPh at http://www.globalrph.com/medterm6b.htm, which defines itself as The Clinician's Ultimate Reference, tells us this simply means left. Now how did I miss that when I studied Greek and Latin all those years ago? Looks like my spine curves outward to the left. I couldn't find any relationship between this and CKD except that it may cause kidney pain if the curvature is severe enough.

Sure enough, there is a connection between CKD and the spurring of my thoracic spine and it's degeneration. But wait. I forget to explain spurring. This is how it was explained in *The Book of Blogs: Moderate Stage Chronic Kidney Disease, Part 2*:

"...bone spur. A what? Oh, an osteophyte! Osteo comes from the Latin *osseus*—*os*, *ossis* meaning bone and the Greek *osteon*, also meaning bone. {Thank you for the memory, Hunter College of the City University of New York course in Greek and Latin roots taken a zillion years ago.}"

Funny how the memory works sometimes and others it doesn't. I can just see one of my kids rolling her eyes and saying, "So?" So, it means that there is extra bone growing on my poor thoracic spine as part of the degeneration of my body. Even though it's my body I'm writing about, I find it amusing that bone is growing rather than diminishing as part of the degeneration. It seems backwards to me.

However, there you have it: chronic kidney disease is a degenerative disease. The spurring of the thoracic spine is also degenerative. Since I just turned 70, I'm not surprised about the spine thing. Keep in mind that CKD can hit at any age.

You knew it. This is turning into a plea to get tested for CKD. Here's a bit of information from the National Kidney Foundation of Arizona that can help with that:

"Path to Wellness screenings provide free blood and urine testing, which is evaluated onsite is using point-of-care testing devices to assess for the risk of diabetes, heart and kidney diseases. Those screened are also presented with chronic disease management education, an overall health assessment (weight, blood pressure, etc.) and a one-on-one consultation with a physician. Enrollment opportunities are offered for a follow-up 6-week series of Healthy Living workshops that teach chronic disease self-management skills. For more information, click the link above or call our main line at: (602) 840-1644."

2/10/17 *At Last: Cuba*

I've been saying for a couple of weeks now that I would write about Cuba, or rather The Republic of Cuba since that is the country's official title. That's where I spent my Groundhog's Day 70th birthday in the company of my husband, brother, and sister-in-law. By the way, whenever we travel together, they are the best part of the trip no matter what we see or where we go.

But I digress; Cuba is a beautiful country with friendly people and colorful buildings painted in those colors the government approves ... in addition to free education and free medical care. Considering Cuba is a country run by The Communist Party, maybe this universal medical and education isn't as free as we might think.

Let's take a look at the education first since you can't have nephrologists without education. While there is free education, you need to be loyal to the government and perform community service as the 'price' of receiving it. I wasn't clear about how you demonstrated "loyal to the government," but the Cubanos (as the Cuban people refer to themselves) politely declined to discuss this.

The education includes six years of basics of reading, writing, and arithmetic – the same 3 Rs we study in grade school in the USA. After that, there are three years of middle school with traditional school subjects that are taught pretty much anywhere. But then things change. Cubanos can attend what we might consider a traditional high school for three years or a vocational school for three years. This is also when marching in parades and community service begins.

Nephrologists would have chosen the traditional high school. After that, there's another five to six years of university for their medical degree. Not everyone attends university; students need to pass certain exams in order to be allowed to attend… something we're used to hearing. So now our doctor has become a doctor. What additional education is needed to become a nephrologist?

I tried to question the people I met in ports of call, but again they declined to answer in full. From the little bit I got from them and the even less I could garner from the internet: all medical students need to do a residency in General Medicine. If you want to go on to a specialty – like Nephrology – you need to do an additional residency in that field.

Well, what about the medicine itself? What do Cubano doctors know about nephrology?

According to Radio Angulo – Cuba's information radio – on November 23 of last year,

"The positive development of this specialty began with the triumph of the Revolution in 1959, as Dr. Charles Magrans Buch, full professor and professor emeritus, told Granma International. Magrans began practicing his profession in 1958 in the Clinico de 26, today the Joaquin Albarran Clinical-Surgical Teaching Hospital, home to the Dr. Abelardo Buch Lopez Institute of Nephrology."

Granma International describes itself as The Official Voice of the Communist Party of Cuba Central Committee.

As for the quality of the medical schools,

"…Cuba trains young physicians worldwide in its Latin American School of Medicine (ELAM). Since its inception in 1998, ELAM has graduated more than 20,000 doctors from over 123 countries.

Currently, 11,000 young people from over 120 nations follow a career in medicine at the Cuban institution."

You can read more about ELAM in Salim Lamrani's blog in the 8/8/14 edition of The Huffington Post at http://www.huffingtonpost.com/salim-lamrani/cubas-health-care-system-_b_5649968.html

Yesterday, I stumbled upon this which is also from Granma:

"The Cuban Institute of Nephrology is celebrating its 50th anniversary this December 1st, having provided more than 5,000 kidney transplants and 3,125 patients with dialysis."

So, nephrology is not new to Cuba nor is there a dearth of opportunities to study this specialty. Keep in mind that this is government run health care. There aren't any private clinics or hospitals in Cuba.

And how good is that health care system? This is from the 4/9/14 HavanaTimes.org:

"Boasting health statistics above all other countries in Latin America and the Caribbean (and even the United States), Cuba's healthcare system has achieved world recognition and been endorsed by the World and Pan-American Health Organizations and the United Nations."

HavanaTimes.org is not part of the government. Some of their writers have been blacklisted, while others have been questioned. Somehow, that makes me feel more secure that their information is not the party line but more truthful. I don't mean to say the government is dishonest, but I prefer information from private sources in this case.

Before you get your passport in order and book a trip to Cuba for medical reasons, you should know

"…it is not legal for Americans to go to Cuba as medical tourists…."

This information is from Cuba Medical Travel Adviser & Guide at http://www.doctorcuba.com/.

What I found curious is that it is not illegal for Cuban doctors to treat American patients in Cuba. Do Americans disguise themselves as being from other countries to obtain the low cost, high quality medical treatment Cuba has to offer? How can they do that if a passport is needed to enter the country? Maybe I'm naïve.

Cuban medicine follows a different model than that of the USA. A general (family) doctor earns about $20 a month with free housing and food. His or her mornings are spent at the clinic with the afternoons reserved for house calls. Doctors treat patients and/or research. Preventive medicine is the norm with shortages of medication and supplies a constant problem.

You have to remember that I have limited access to information about Cuba (as does the rest of the world), and am not so certain my even more limited Spanish – which is not even Cubano Spanish – and the limited English of the Cubanos I spoke with has allowed me to fully understand the answers I was given to the questions I asked.

It's been fun sharing what I think I learned with you since it brought the feeling of being in Cuba right back. Can you hear the music? I've got to get up to dance.

2/27/17 *February is Black History Month*

In honor of Black History Month, I thought I would write about Blacks who have contributed to the research and treatment of Chronic Kidney Disease. I'll be highlighting a few people and then dealing with why CKD is treated differently for Blacks.

Ladies first: Dr. Bessie Young is a nephrologist... and more. This is from The University of Washington's Department of Medicine at https://medicine.uw.edu/news/dr-bessie-young.

"Dr. Young is a professor of medicine in the Division of Nephrology and holds adjunct titles in the Departments of Epidemiology and Health Services. She received her MD in 1987 and her MPH in 2001, both from the University of Washington.

Her research focuses on racial disparities and genetic factors predicting outcomes of patients with kidney disease, education regarding access to transplantation and dialysis for minorities, and access to kidney disease care in rural areas."

While I have great admiration for both Drs. Young and Kountz (see below), I feel a connection with Dr. Vanessa Grubbs. We corresponded a bit when she first began her blog, which is both personal and professional. We all know I'm not a doctor and have never claimed to be one, but I'm convinced I can feel what a nephrologist feels when I read her blog. This is from The California Health Care Foundation's website:

"Dr. Grubbs is an assistant professor of medicine in the Division of Nephrology at the University of California, San Francisco, Zuckerberg San Francisco General Hospital, where she has maintained a clinical practice and clinical research program since 2009. Though most of her time is dedicated to research and patient care, her passion is creative nonfiction writing. She is working on her first book, and she blogs at thenephrologist.com."

Her book, *Hundreds of Interlaced Fingers: A Kidney Doctor's Search for the Perfect Match* will be available on Amazon.com this June. By the way, she donated a kidney to her husband when they were only dating.

Samuel L. Kountz, M.D was another innovative contributor to Nephrology from the Black Community. As Blackpast.org tells us:

"In 1961 Kountz and Roy Cohn, another leading surgeon, performed the first successful kidney transplant between two people who were close relatives but not twins. Over the next decade Kountz researched the process of kidney transplants on dogs. He discovered that monitoring blood flow into the new kidney and administering methylprednisolone to the patient after surgery allowed the body to accept the new organ.

In 1966 Kountz joined the faculty at Stanford University Hospital and Medical School and in 1967 he became the chief of the kidney transplant service at University of California at San Francisco (UCSF). There he worked with Folker Belzer to create the Belzer kidney perfusion machine. This innovation kept kidneys alive for 50 hours after being removed from the donor. Through Kountz's involvement at UCSF, the institution's kidney transplant research center became one the best in the country. Kountz also created the Center for Human Values at UCSF, to discuss ethical issues concerning transplants."

It's time for an explanation as to why I wrote "why CKD is treated differently for Blacks," isn't it?

This is from Jane E. Brody's article *Doctors sharpen message on kidney disease* reprinted in **The Book of Blogs: Moderate Stage Chronic Kidney Disease, Part 1**:

"There are four main risk factors for kidney disease: diabetes, high blood pressure, age over 60 and a family history of the disease. Anyone with these risk factors should have a test of kidney function at least once a year, Vassalotti said. (Me here: he was the National Kidney Foundation's Chief Medical Officer at the time the article was written). Members of certain ethnic groups are also at higher than average risk: blacks, Hispanics, Pacific Islanders and Native Americans."

This means physicians need to monitor blood pressure and diabetes more closely for blacks (as well as the other high risk groups). Why, you ask. This bit from **What Is It and How Did I Get It? Early Stage Chronic Kidney Disease** will explain about the blood pressure.

"HPB can damage small blood vessels in the kidneys to the point that they cannot filter the waste from the blood as effectively as they should. Nephrologists may prescribe HBP medication to prevent your CKD from getting worse since these medications reduce the amount of protein in your urine. Not too surprisingly, most CKD related deaths are caused by cardiovascular problems."

As for diabetes, I turned to **The Book of Blogs: Moderate Chronic Kidney Disease, Part 2**, for this tidbit:

"According to Diabetes.co.uk at http://www.diabetes.co.uk/how-does-diabetes-affect-the-body.html, 'The kidneys are another organ that is at particular risk of damage as a result of diabetes and the risk is again increased by poorly controlled diabetes, high blood pressure and cholesterol'"

In addition, there is a gene more prevalent in Blacks that can exacerbate their CKD. "This discovery provides direct evidence that African-Americans with established CKD and the APOL1 risk gene variant experience a faster decline in kidney function compared to their white counterparts, irrespective in most cases of what caused their kidney disease." Afshin Parsa, M.D., a nephrologist at the University of Maryland School of Medicine in Baltimore and a CRIC Study investigator.

Dr. Parsa was referring to the study on APOL1 which was published in *The New England Journal of Medicine.*
The following is from The National Kidney Foundation's Fact Sheet on Blacks and CKD at https://www.kidney.org/news/newsroom/factsheets/African-Americans-and-CKD.

- Blacks and African Americans suffer from kidney failure at a significantly higher rate than Caucasians – more than 3 times higher.
- African Americans constitute more than 35% of all patients in the U.S. receiving dialysis for kidney failure, but only represent 13.2% of the overall U.S. population.
- Diabetes is the leading cause of kidney failure in African Americans. African Americans are twice as likely to be diagnosed with diabetes as Caucasians. Approximately 4.9 million African Americans over 20 years of age are living with either diagnosed or undiagnosed diabetes.
- The most common type of diabetes in African Americans is type 2 diabetes. The risk factors for this type of diabetes include: family history, impaired glucose tolerance, diabetes during pregnancy, hyperinsulinemia and insulin resistance, obesity and physical inactivity. African Americans with diabetes are more likely to develop complications of diabetes and to have greater disability from these complications than Caucasians. African Americans are also more

likely to develop serious complications such as heart disease and strokes.

- High blood pressure is the second leading cause of kidney failure among African Americans, and remains the leading cause of death due to its link with heart attacks and strokes.
-

Today's blog was a bit longer than usual to bring you this important information. We celebrate Black History Month AND need to make our Black family members, friends, and co-workers aware of their heightened risk so they can help prevent their own CKD.

3/6/17 *Women and Water (Men, too)*

Welcome to March: National Kidney Month and Women's History Month. I'm going to fudge a bit on the 'History' part of that as I did last month with Black History Month. I don't often have guest bloggers, but this month will feature two women as guest bloggers in honor of Women's History Month.

The first is Jessica Walter, who sent me the following email last month:

Hi There,
I am a freelance health and food writer, I have teamed up with a small senior lifestyle advice site, I worked with them to develop a complete guide on how to eat better and be healthier from a dietary point of view. This includes detailed information on why being hydrated is so important. ... you can check out the article here: https://www.senioradvisor.com/ blog/2017/02/7-tips-on- developing-better-eating- habits-in-your-senior-years/.

I liked what Jessica had to say and how easily it could be adapted not only for senior Chronic Kidney Disease patients, but all Chronic Kidney Disease patients.

In addition, she sent me this short article about hydration and CKD. It's easy to read and has some information we constantly need to be reminded of.

Staying Hydrated When You Have Chronic Kidney Disease
We all know that drinking water is important for our health, and monitoring fluid intake is critical for those with chronic kidney disease. Too much water can be problematic, but so can too little. Dehydration can be serious for those with chronic kidney disease. If you are suffering from vomiting, diarrhea, fever, or diabetes, or if you urinate frequently, you may become dehydrated be-

cause you are losing more fluid than you are taking in. For those without chronic kidney disease, the solution is to increase the intake of water until the body is sufficiently hydrated.

Since dehydration can decrease blood flow to the kidneys, and as fluid intake must be controlled in patients with chronic kidney disease, it's important to closely monitor their fluid intake and loss in these circumstances.

Recognizing The Signs

The first step is to recognize the physical signs of dehydration. You may have a dry mouth or dry eyes, heart palpitations, muscle cramps, lightheadedness or fainting, nausea, or vomiting. You may notice a decrease in your urine output. Weight loss of more than a pound or two over a few days can also be an indicator of dehydration. If you are taking ACE inhibitors and ARBs, such as lisinopril, enalapril, valsartan, or losartan, or water pills or diuretics, these medications can harm your kidneys if you become dehydrated. It is doubly important to be aware of signs of dehydration if you are on any of these medications.

Steps to Take

To rehydrate your body, start by increasing your intake of water and ensure that you are eating plenty of fruits and vegetables. (Me here: remember to stay within your renal diet guidelines for fruits, vegetables, and fluids.)If you cannot keep water down, or if increased consumption doesn't alleviate the signs of dehydration, contact your health care provider immediately. They may also recommend a different fluid than plain water since electrolytes and minerals can also be reduced if you are dehydrated, but you may still need to watch your intake of potassium, phosphorus, protein, and sodium. Your doctor may recommend an oral rehydration solution that will restore your body to a proper level of hydration. If you have a fluid restriction because you are on dialysis, you should consult your healthcare provider if you have issues with or questions about hydration. Taking in or retaining too much fluid when you have these restrictions can lead to serious complications, including headaches, swelling, high blood pressure and even stroke. Carefully monitoring your fluid intake and watching for signs of dehydration will help you to avoid the consequences of dehydration.

I've blogged many times over the last six years about hydration. I'm enjoying reading this important material from another's point of view. I'm sorry Jessica's grandmother had to suffer this, but I'm also glad Jessica chose to share her writing about it with us.

This June, 2010, article included in *The Book of Blogs: Moderate Chronic Kidney Disease, Part 1* furthers explains:

"....Dr. HL Trivedi of the Institute of Kidney Diseases and Research Centre (IKDRC) said, '.... Rapid water loss causes the kidney's functioning to slow down, resulting in temporary or permanent kidney failure.'

Extreme heat causes rapid water loss, resulting in acute electrolyte imbalance. The kidney, unable to cope with the water loss, fails to flush out the requisite amount of Creatinine and other toxins from the body. Coupled with a lack of consistent water intake, this brings about permanent or temporary kidney failure, explain experts."

The article can be viewed directly at http://www.dnaindia.com/health/report_heat-induced-kidney-ailments-see-40pct-rise_1390589 and is from "Daily News & Analysis."

The CDC also offers advice to avoid heat illness:

"People with a chronic medical condition are less likely to sense and respond to changes in temperature. Also, they may be taking medications that can worsen the impact of extreme heat. People in this category need the following information.

- Drink more water than usual and don't wait until you're thirsty to drink.
- Check on a friend or neighbor, and have someone do the same for you.
- Check the local news for health and safety updates regularly.
- Don't use the stove or oven to cook——it will make you and your house hotter.
- Wear loose, lightweight, light-colored clothing.
- Take cool showers or baths to cool down.
- Seek medical care immediately if you or someone you know experiences symptoms of heat-related illness (http://www.cdc.gov/extremeheat/warning)

It's clear we need to keep an eye on our hydration.

3/13/17 *Processed Foods: Yea or Nay?*

Good morning, world! It's still March which means it's still National Kidney Month here in the USA and Women's History Month. I'm going to take liberties with the 'history' part of Women's History Month just as I did last month with Black History Month. Today we have a guest blog from a woman – Diana Mrozek, RDN – which deals with the kidneys.

You know you're entitled to a free nutritional appointment yearly after two the first year if you have CKD. Here's what I wrote about that in **What Is It and How Did I Get It? Early Stage Chronic Kidney Disease:**

"Most people think of a nutritionist as a luxury even if they do have a chronic disease. When I pulled out my checkbook to pay my renal dietitian [RD], I was told the government will pay for her services. That made sense. Especially in the current economic atmosphere and for older people, the government needs to help pay our medical bills."

My nephrologist is part of a practice which rotates their nutritionists. It's a pretty good idea since I get different points of view about my renal diet from dietitians who each have my records at hand. Your renal diet is tweaked according to your latest labs, so having your records in front of them is important to you and your nutritionist.

Notice I was writing about a RD and Diana is a RDN. The only difference between the two is that Registered Dieticians need not also be Nutritionists, but an RDN is both a Dietician and a Nutritionist.

Let's take a look at Diana's unique take on processed foods now.
Processed Food, Chronic Kidney Disease and Your Health

What foods come to mind when you hear the words "processed food"? Is it potato chips? Fast food? Margarine? Or maybe bread? Olive oil? Milk? Do you think artificial? Unhealthy? Safe? Convenient? Cheap?

If any of these words or foods came to mind, you are correct! Let's clarify. Processed is a term that applies to a wide range of foods as by definition they are any food that has been altered from its natural state usually for either safety or convenience. Many foods need to be processed to make them suitable for eating, for example extracting oil from seeds and pasteurizing milk to make it safe to drink.

Processed foods can have many benefits like convenient and safe food storage as well as better retention of nutrient content. For example, flash frozen fruits and vegetables may have higher vitamin and mineral content than fresh or canned. They also provide more choice, less waste, less cost and can reduce food preparation and cooking time. Processed foods can be helpful for people who have difficulty cooking, like the elderly or disabled.

Over the past several years, many working in the nutrition industry have become very critical of processed foods, and their widespread use in our diet has been blamed for everything from obesity to cancer. However, other than fresh produce straight from the fields, you would have a hard time finding many unprocessed foods in your local grocery store. Most store-bought foods have been processed in some way including freezing, canning, baking, drying, irradiating and pasteurizing. Processed foods are here to stay, but making informed choices when grocery shopping will allow them to be part of a healthy, balanced diet.

The problem with some of today's processed foods are the amounts of salt, sugar and fat that are often added to enhance taste, extend shelf life and retain moisture, texture, etc. Because we rely heavily on processed foods, we may be eating more salt, sugar and fat than we need. This is important for people with kidney disease who need to watch salt intake for blood pressure control. Kidney patients who also have diabetes need to limit sugar intake as well. Since both diabetes and kidney disease increase the risk of heart disease, fat intake is another concern.

So how do you select healthier processed foods? In general, you want to choose products with less fat and sodium, more fiber and the least added sugar. The best way to do this is to read the Nutrition Facts Label and stick to eating one serving of packaged foods. Use the following guidelines when looking at different nutrients and ingredients on the nutrition labels to make better choices:

Trans Fats – Look for 0 grams. Trans fats are hidden in many fried and baked foods like biscuits, cookies, crackers as well as frozen foods. They increase levels of bad cholesterol (LDL) and decrease good cholesterol (HDL). If you see shortening or partially hydrogenated oils in the ingredient list, it has trans fat. Remember...Trans fat? Put it back!

Saturated fat – For most people, intake of saturated fat should be around 13-18 grams per day.

Sodium – Sodium intake should be less than 2300 milligrams (mg) per day or 700-800 mg per meal. Look for "no salt added" canned items or items with preferably less than 200 mg per serving. Limit use of boxed side dishes with seasoning packets as well as high sodium condiments like soy sauce, barbeque sauce and bottled dressing and marinades.

Sugar – Sugars are a bit trickier. Instead of grams, check ingredient lists for sugars like corn sweetener and high fructose corn syrup, and words ending in -ose, like dextrose or maltose. If a sugar ingredient is one of the first three ingredients in the list or if there are more than 2-3 different types of sugars, it likely has a lot of added sugar.

Fiber – Look for at least 3 grams of fiber per serving for cereal, bread and crackers. Also, look for the word "whole" before grains, like whole wheat. If it says enriched, it's likely had the fiber removed during processing.

By spending a few extra minutes of your shopping time taking a closer look at the groceries you are buying, you can limit less healthy additives and still enjoy all the benefits of processed foods!

While I agree with Diana now that she's brought up processed foods, remember your labs will dictate your renal diet.

3/20/17 *Women Marching to the Kidney's Beat*

In keeping with my theme of March being Women's History Month – minus the history – and National Kidney Month, today's blog will be about those women around the world who have contributed to Chronic Kidney Disease knowledge. Two such women, Dr. Vanessa Grubbs and Dr. Bessie Young, were highlighted in February's tribute to Black History Month and women in nephrology. Thank you again, ladies, for all you do for CKD patients.

When you realize the study of nephrology as we know it is only a little over 50 years old (Incredible, isn't it?), you'll understand why I raided The International Society of Nephrologists (ISN) October 2010 issue for the following information. I've added notes for clarification when needed.

United States: An accomplished researcher and physician, Josephine Briggs is a former ISN councilor and former councilor and Secretary of ASN (American Society of Nephrologists). She is the former director of the Division of Kidney, Urologic, and Hematologic Diseases, National Institute of Diabetes and Digestive and Kidney Diseases (NIDDK), US National Institutes of Health (NIH), and was responsible for all NIH funded renal research in the 1990s. Today, she is Director of the National Center for Complementary and Alternative Medicine. She maintains a lab at NIDDK, researching the renin-angiotensin system, diabetic nephropathy, circadian regulation of blood pressure, and the effect of antioxidants in kidney disease.

Europe: Rene Habib, who passed away (in 2010), was a truly pioneering renal pathologist. She provided the first description of many renal diseases and worked with ISN founder Jean Hamburger to establish nephrology as a new discipline in Europe. Her contributions and energy were central to establishing pathology as an essential and integrated component of this new field worldwide.

45

India: Vidya N. Acharya was the first woman nephrologist in India and trained some 150 internists in nephrology. For three decades, her research focused on Urinary Tract Infection. She was a consultant nephrologist at Gopalakrishna Piramal Memorial Hospital and director of the Piramal Institute for training in Dialysis Technology, Renal Nutrition and Preventive Nephrology in Mumbai. She received a Lifetime Achievement Award from the Indian Society of Nephrology in 2007.

China: HaiYan Wang is the Editor of Kidney International China and has been an ISN and ASPN (American Society of Pediatric Nephrology) councilor and Executive Committee member as well as a member of the editorial boards of Chinese and international renal journals. She has published over 200 articles and books in Chinese and English. She graduated from Beijing Medical University. After three years of internship, she became a nephrology fellow at the First Hospital Beijing Medical University. Since 1983, she moved on to Chief of Nephrology and later became Professor of the Department of Medicine at the First Hospital Beijing. She has been Chairman of the Chinese Society of Nephrology and is Vice President of the Chinese Medical Association. Her unit is the largest training site for nephrology fellows in China.

United Arab Emirates: Mona Alrukhaimi is co-chair of the ISN GO (International Society of Nephrologists Global Outreach Programs) Middle East Committee, and the leader of the KDIGO (Kidney Disease: Improving Global Outcomes) Implementation Task Force for the Middle East and African regions. She is also a Member of the Governing Board of the Arab Society of Nephrology and Renal Transplantation. Since 2006, she has actively organized World Kidney Day activities in the United Arab Emirates and prepared the past four rounds of the ISN Update Course in Nephrology. Having played an active role in the Declaration of Istanbul on Organ Trafficking and Transplant Tourism, she contributes to serve on the custodian group and takes part in the Steering Committee for Women in Transplantation under The Transplantation Society.

South Africa: Saraladevi Naicker carried the weight of setting standards and provided the first training program for nephrologists in Africa over the last decade (Remember this article was published in 2010.). Specializing in internal medicine, she trained in Durban and later helped set up a Transplant Unit in the Renal Unit at Addington Hospital. In 2001, she became Chief Specialist and Professor of Renal Medicine at University of Witwatersrand in Johannesburg and in 2009 was appointed Chairman of Medicine at Wits. She is proud that there are currently (Again: in 2010) six postgraduate students from Africa studying for higher degrees in nephrology under her tutelage. Over the years, Naicker's unit has served as the main training site for young nephrologists from across Africa and many individuals trained by her are currently practicing in Africa. Naicker received the Phillip Tobias Distinguished Teaching Award in 2006, an honor which bears testimony to her teaching prowess.

Israel: Batya Kristal is Professor of Medicine at the Technion Medical School, Haifa. She is the first woman to direct an academic nephrology department in Israel. At the Western Galilee Hospital, Nahariya, she leads a translational research project focusing on different aspects of oxidative stress and inflammation. She also heads a large clinical nephrology and dialysis program, which uniquely integrates staff and patients from the diverse ethnic population of the Galilee. Founder of the Israeli NKF, initiator and organizer of the traditional annual international conferences at Nahariya, she is truly an important role model for women in the country.

Australia: After holding resident positions in medicine and surgery and as registrar in medicine at the Baragwanath Hospital in Johannesburg, Priscilla Kincaid-Smith was director and physician of

Nephrology at Royal Melbourne Hospital and Professor of Medicine at University of Melbourne. She demonstrated overwhelming evidence of the link between headache powders and kidney damage and contributed to research on the links between high blood pressure and renal malfunction. The only female ISN President so far, she was named Commander of the Order of the British Empire "for services to medicine", was awarded the David Hume Award from the National Kidney Foundation (USA) and became a Companion of the Order of Australia.

3/27/17 *Getting Juiced*

I have the gentlest nephrologist in the world! Well, I think so anyway. He has been cautioning me about my weight for years. Yes, there it is again: my weight. Here I was finally coming to terms with being a chubby since nothing I was doing seemed to work to lose the weight. That's when he tossed out a bombshell.

We all know that increased weight can raise your blood pressure which, in turn, negatively affects your kidneys. I was so pleased with myself for having raised my GFR another three points on my last blood test that I didn't understand how I could be leaking protein into my urine at the same time. Wasn't protein in the urine simply an indication that you have Chronic Kidney Disease? Didn't I already know that? So why was protein leaking into my urine to the tune of 252 mg. when the norm was between 15-220 mg?

I know, I know: back up a bit. Thanks for the reminder. GFR is defined in **What Is It and How Did I Get It? Early Stage Chronic Kidney Disease** this way:

"GFR: Glomerular filtration rate [if there is a lower case 'e' before the term, it means estimated glomerular filtration rate] which determines both the stage of kidney disease and how well the kidneys are functioning."

Oh, and just in case you've forgotten, this excerpt from **The Book of Blogs: Moderate Stage Chronic Kidney Disease, Part 2** is a good reminder about the stages of CKD.

"Different stages require different treatment or no treatment at all. There are five stages with the mid-level stage divided into two parts. The higher the stage, the worse your kidney function. Think of the stages as a test with 100 being the highest score. These are the stages and their treatments:

STAGE 1: (normal or high) – above 90 – usually requires watching, not treatment, although many people decide to make life style changes now: following a renal diet, exercising, lowering blood pressure, ceasing to smoke, etc.

STAGE 2: (mild) – 60-89 – Same as for stage one

STAGE 3A: (moderate) – 45-59 – This is when you are usually referred to a nephrologist [Kidney specialist]. You'll need a renal [Kidney] dietitian, too, since you need to be rigorous in avoiding more than certain amounts of protein, potassium, phosphorous, and sodium in your diet to slow down the deterioration of your kidneys. Each patient has different needs so there is no one diet. The diet is based on your lab results. Medications such as those for high blood pressure may be prescribed to help preserve your kidney function.

STAGE 3B: (moderate) – 30-44 – same as above, except the patient may experience symptoms.

STAGE 4: (severe 15-29) – Here's when dialysis may start. A kidney transplant may be necessary instead of dialysis [Artificial cleansing of your blood]. Your nephrologist will probably want to see you every three months and request labs before each visit.

STAGE 5: (End stage) – below 15 – Dialysis or transplant is necessary to continue living.

Many thanks to DaVita for refreshing my memory about each stage."

Okay, back to the connection between spilling protein into your urine (called proteinuria) and CKD. This is from *SlowItDownCKD 2016*:

"In *The Book of Blogs: Moderate Chronic Kidney Disease, Part 1*, The National Institutes of Health helped me explain why this combination of excess weight and pre-diabetes was a problem for CKD patients:

'High blood glucose and high blood pressure damage the kidneys' filters. When the kidneys are damaged, proteins leak out of the kidneys into the urine. The urinary albumin test detects this loss of protein in the urine. Damaged kidneys do not do a good job of filtering out wastes and extra fluid. Wastes and fluid build up in your blood instead of leaving the body in urine.'"

Let's say you don't have pre-diabetes, but do have CKD. Does proteinuria still make it worse? Damn! It does. This explanation is from *SlowItDownCKD 2015*:

"The problem is that antibodies are made up of protein. Antibodies is defined by Dictionary.com at http://dictionary.reference.com/browse/antibodies as

'A protein substance produced in the blood or tissues in response to a specific antigen, such as a bacterium or a toxin, that destroys or weakens bacteria and neutralizes organic poisons, thus forming the basis of immunity.'

Lose lots of protein into your urine and you're losing some of your immunity. In other words, you're open to infection."

I guess that explains why I magically developed a UTI after years of not having any.

I have gone so far afield from what I intended to write about on this last Monday of National Kidney Month. What was that, you ask? It was my nephrologist's strong suggestions for immediate weight loss: juicing. I was so surprised.

After all that writing about eating the raw vegetables for roughage and sticking to only three specified amount servings of each daily, this expert in his field was telling me to ignore all that and throw myself into juicing for the immediate future. But you can bet I'll try it; no way I'm throwing nine years of keeping my kidneys healthier and healthier out the window.

I can't tell you if it works since I only started yesterday, but I can tell you it doesn't taste bad. I'm learning how to use this fancy-dancy blender we got three years ago that had just been sitting on the shelf. Experimenting with the consistency has caused a mess here and there, but oh well.

My first juicing experience included kale, celery, lemons, cucumbers, and ginger. I definitely need to play with my combinations. I also think I made far too much. Luckily Bear was in the house and shouted out that the machine was making that noise because I didn't add enough water. Water? You're supposed to add water?

I'll keep you posted on these experiments if you'll get yourself tested for CKD. It's just a blood and urine test. Fair deal?

4/3/17 *Just Blend In*

Well, if that doesn't beat all! Here I thought I was juicing until a reader asked me if my nephrologist knew the difference between juicing and blending. There's something called blending? Let's get my doctor out of the equation right away. He may or may not know the difference between the two, but I certainly didn't.

I heard juicing and just assumed (and we all know what happens when we assume) it meant tossing 80% vegetables – since this was prescribed for fast weight loss – and 20% fruits in the blender. Hmmm, the name of the machine I used should have tipped me off that there was a difference, but it went right over my head. Let me tell you what I learned. Juice, according to Dictionary.com at http://www.dictionary.com/browse/juicing, is:

"the natural fluid, fluid content or liquid part that can be extracted from a plant or one of its parts..."

while juicing is
"to extract juice from."

Uh-uh, I wasn't doing that. There was no pulp left after the vegetables and fruits were processed in the blender. It all sort of mushed – oh, all right – blended together.

The same dictionary tells me blending is:

"to mix smoothly and inseparably together."

Yep, that's what I've been doing. By the way, for those of you who asked to be kept posted about any weight loss, I've lost five pounds in ten days. To be perfectly candid, there was one day of I'm-going-to-eat-anything-I –want! mixed in there.

Another CKD Awareness Advocate wondered just what I was doing to my electrolyte limits while on this blending (I do know that's what it is now.) diet. I arbitrarily chose a recipe from a juicing book I got online before I realized I wasn't juicing. The recipe called for:

2 beets (what a mess to peel and chop)
2 carrots (I used the equivalent in baby ones since my hands were already starting to hurt from dealing with the beets)
8 strawberries
7 leaves of kale – which I learned is also called Tuscan cabbage
I added a cup of water since I wasn't taking any pulp out, so the mixture was really thick.

All the ingredients were on my renal diet. So far, so good. But the question was about my daily electrolyte limits. My limits are as follows (Yours may be different since the limits usually are based upon your most current labs.):

Calories – 2100
Potassium – 3000 mg.
Phosphorous – 800 mg.
Protein – 5 ounces (141,748 mg.)
Sodium – 2000 mg.

Nutritional Data at http://nutritiondata.self.com/facts/vegetables-and-vegetable-products/2348/2 tells me I drank this much of each of those electrolytes in the total of two drinks I had of this concoction... I mean blend. The measurement is milligrams and each drink replaces a meal.

	Protein	Phosphorus
Beets	1300	33
Carrots	2700	42
Kale	2200	38

Strawberries	1000	37
Totals	7200	150

	Potassium	Sodium
Beets	267	1300
Carrots	359	2700
Kale	299	2200
Strawberries	233	1000
Totals	1158	7200

	Calories
Beets	33
Carrots	42
Kale	38
Strawberries	37
Totals	150

I had to backtrack a little to figure out that 8 baby carrots is the equivalent to 2/3 of a cup or a little over five oz. Thanks to http://www.fruitsandveggiesmorematters.org/how-much-do-i-need for the help there. They were also the source I used to verify that 8 large strawberries equal 1 cup or 8 oz.

The calculations were the hardest part of this blog for me. I rounded up whenever possible. Also, keep in mind that different sites or books may give you different approximations for the electrolytes in the different amounts of each different food you blend. I discovered that when I was researching and decided to stick with the simplest site for me to understand.

So, did I exceed my limits? I am permitted three different vegetables per day with a serving of half a cup per vegetable. There are
only three vegetables in this recipe. I did go over ½ cup with the
all of them, yet am under my limitations for each of the electrolytes. This is complicated. As for the fruit, I am also allowed three
different ones with ½ cup limit on each. Or can I count the one
cup of strawberries as two servings of today's vegetables? Welcome to my daily conundrum.

Over all, I still have plenty of electrolytes available to me for my
third meal today, which is to be a light meal of regular foods (provided they're on my renal diet). I also have two cups of coffee a
day which has its own numbers:

Protein	Phosphorus	Potassium	Sodium	Calories
6000	14	232	9	4

Add those in and I still have plenty of food available to me with
the electrolytes within the balance limits. The funny part is that
I'm not hungry for hours after one of the blended drinks and,
bam! all of a sudden I'm ravenous. I usually have the light meal
mid-day so I'm not still digesting at bedtime. This is really important: on that I'm-going-to-eat-anything-I –want! day, I was
hungrier and hungrier the more I ate and didn't recognize when I
was full.

The nice part about blending is that the fiber is still in the mixture.
Fiber is necessary for a multitude of reasons when you're a CKD
patient. DaVita at https://www.davita.com/kidney-disease/diet-
and-nutrition/diet-basics/fiber-in-the-kidney-diet/e/5320 lists
those reasons for us:

Benefits of fiber
Adequate fiber in the kidney diet can be beneficial to people with
chronic kidney disease (CKD) because it:

- Keeps GI (gastrointestinal) function healthy
- Adds bulk to stool to prevent constipation
- Prevents diverticulosis (pockets inside the colon)
- Helps increase water in stool for easier bowel movements
- Promotes regularity
- Prevents hemorrhoids
- Helps control blood sugar and cholesterol

4/10/17 *The Helper Asks for Help*

Imagine my surprise when I received an email from Deanna Power, Director of Outreach Disability Benefits Help at the Social Security Administration. My first thought: are they raising my monthly amount? But isn't it the wrong time of year for an awards letter from them? And why would the email be from Disability anyway? Hmmm, so I did the logic thing; I opened the email and read it.

Look at this! Ms. Power wants me to help those on dialysis and those who have a transplant understand the application for SSA. While I don't usually deal with either End Stage Chronic Kidney Disease or Transplantation, this struck me as worthwhile. Take note of the possibility of SSA for less advanced kidney disease, too. So, without further ado...

■■

If you have been diagnosed with kidney disease, you know that maintaining your career can be challenging due to your health needs and frequent doctor's appointments. There might be financial assistance available for you.

The Social Security Administration (SSA) will compare any applicant with kidney disease to its own medical guide of qualifying conditions, the Blue Book (written for medical professionals), which outlines exactly what treatments or test results are needed to qualify. This is under Section 6.00 which outlines three separate listings for kidney disease. Meeting one is enough to medically qualify.

6.03: *Chronic kidney disease with hemodialysis or peritoneal dialysis*. Dialysis must be expected to last for a continuous period of at least one year. Disability benefits will be paid throughout your treatments. An acceptable medical source (blood work, physician's notes, etc.) is needed to approve your claim. You also may meet a kidney disease listing before your first round of dialysis, so be sure to check listing 6.05 (below) if your doctor is considering dialysis.

6.04: *Chronic kidney disease with transplant.* You will automatically medically qualify for disability benefits for at least one year. After that the SSA will reevaluate your claim to determine if you are still eligible for disability benefits.

6.05: *Chronic kidney disease, with impairment of function.* This is the most complicated listing. The Blue Book – which was written for medical professionals – is available online, so you should review it with your doctor to know if you'll qualify. In simplified terms, the Blue Book states:

You must have one of the following lab findings documented on at least two occasions, 90 days apart, within the same year:

- Serum creatinine of 4mg/dL or greater, OR
- Creatinine clearance of 20 ml/min or less, OR
- Estimated glomerular filtration rate of 20 ml/min/1.73m2 or less

Additionally, you must have *one* of the following:
1. Renal osteodystrophy (bone disease caused by kidney failure) with severe bone pain and acceptable imaging documenting bone abnormalities, such as osteitis fibrosa, osteomalacia, or bone fractures, OR
2. Peripheral neuropathy, OR
3. Anorexia with weight loss, determined with a BMI of 18.0 or less, calculated on at least two occasions at least 90 days apart within the same year, OR
4. Fluid overload syndrome with one of the following:

- High blood pressure of 110 Hg despite at least 90 days of taking prescribed medication. Blood pressure must be taken at least 90 days apart during the same year.
- Signs of vascular congestion or anasarca (fluid buildup) despite 90 straight days of prescribed medication. Again, the vascular congestion or anasarca must have been recorded at the hospital at least twice, three months apart, and all within the same year.

You may need additional tests to evaluate your kidney function to determine your eligibility.

The SSA has a special approval process called a "Medical Vocational Allowance" that helps people with less advanced kidney disease get financial assistance when your kidney disease prevents you from performing any work *that you're qualified for.* The SSA will look at how your treatments prevent you from working, and then compare your restrictions to your age, education, and work history.

Older applicants have an easier time qualifying this way, as the SSA believes they'll have a harder time getting retrained for a new job. If you don't have a college degree, you'll also have an easier time getting approved, as people with college degrees often have a variety of skills that can be used at sedentary jobs. The more physical your past jobs, the better your chances of approval. A Medical Vocational Allowance relies heavily on the findings from the Residual Functional Capacity (RFC) evaluation. An RFC documents how much you can stay seated or on your feet, how much weight you can lift, your ability to stoop and walk, and more. You can download an RFC online for your doctor to fill out on your behalf.

The majority of applicants can complete the entire process online. This is the easiest way to apply as you can save your progress to complete your application later. If you'd prefer to apply in person, call the SSA at 1-800-772-1213 to schedule an appointment at your closest Social Security office. There are at least four locations in every state.

The most important components of your application will be your thoroughness and attention to detail. Fill out *every* question on the application. Describe how your kidney disease impacts your ability to work specifically, or how it keeps you from performing daily tasks as you used to. Any complications or side effects from your treatments and medications need to be recorded as well. The SSA will not require you to submit your medical records yourself, but you do need to list every hospital where you've received treatment. If the SSA can't find evidence documenting your kidney disease, you won't be approved.

It takes an average of five months to be approved. That's when your benefits start. You will be eligible for Medicare 24 months after "the onset of your disability," which is typically the point at which your kidney disease stopped you from working. If your kidney disease is end stage, your waiting period will be waived.

∎∎

Many thanks to Ms. Power for suggesting I pass on this information. Please use the links, file your papers, and make life a bit easier for yourself if you fit into any of these designations. It's all about helping each other after all, isn't it?

4/17/17 *Yet Another Possibility*

Today we have yet another fitness plan? Weight loss plan? Health plan? Beauty plan? I don't know what to call it since they offer so many different types of products. What's that, you ask. It's called Wakaya Perfection. It seems a great number of my friends and acquaintances have been involved in their health in this way recently. They, however, do not have Chronic Kidney Disease.

Let's get this part out of the way: I want to go there. Yes, there. Wakaya is not only a company, but an island in the South Pacific and it.is.beautiful. Take a look at their website (wakayaperfection.com) so you can see for yourself… but, of course, that's not what this blog is about.

The company has several different lines, so I decided to look at one product from each to evaluate them for CKD patients. Remember, should they not be viable options for CKD patients does not mean they're not viable for those without CKD.

Let's start with the weight loss products since that's what's on my mind lately. That would be the Bula SlimCap. This is what their website has to say about these caps:

"At Wakaya Perfection, when we say all natural, that is exactly what we mean. Our tropical flavors are:

- Sugar Free
- Fat Free
- Gluten Free

And Contain:
- NO Artificial Flavors, Ingredients or Colors, or Monosodium Glutamate (MSG)
- NO Insect or Animal Matter

- NO Growth Hormones
- NO Antibiotics
- NO Herbicides or Pesticide

That sounds great and appeals to me. Wait a minute, natural is good, but what is it that's natural? I couldn't find an ingredient list other than this:

- All Natural Flavors
- Active Ingredients
- Pink Fijian Ginger
- Stevia Reb-A 98%
- Quick Dissolve Blend
-

What makes it a quick dissolve blend? What are the all-natural flavors? What are the active ingredients? Ginger is permissible for CKD patients, but how much ginger is in each cap? And as for Stevia Reb-A 98%, this is a warning I found on New Health Guide at http://www.newhealthguide.org/Stevia-Side-Effects.html: "The FDA has noted that stevia may have a negative impact on the kidneys, reproductive, cardiovascular systems or blood sugar control." Uh-oh, they mentioned our kidneys.

Oh well, that's only one product and maybe there's some other source of ingredients somewhere. Hmmm, I'd want to know what's in a product and how much of each ingredient is in it before I took it, especially with CKD on my plate.

Let's switch to a fitness product. I stayed away from the protein shake meal replacements for the reasons I explained about such products in *SlowItDownCKD 2016*. This is the poignant part of that blog:

"Ladies and gentlemen, our protein intake is restricted because we have CKD. Why would we take a chance on increasing the protein in our bodies? Here's a reminder from *What Is It and How Did I Get It? Early Stage Chronic Kidney Disease* about why we need to limit our protein.

'So, why is protein limited? One reason is that it is the source of a great deal of phosphorus. Another is that a number of nephrons were already destroyed before you were even diagnosed. Logically, those that remain compensate for those that are no longer viable. The remaining nephrons are doing more work than they were meant to. Just like a car that is pushed too hard, there will be constant deterioration if you don't stop pushing. The idea is to stop pushing your remaining nephrons to work even harder in an attempt to slow down the advancement of your CKD. Restricting protein is a way to reduce the nephrons' work.'"

Why don't we take a look at the BulaFit Burn Capsules? Wakaya Perfection describes them as,

"A potent combination of herbs and extracts that help you manage appetite/cravings while providing sustained energy and heightened focus throughout your day. BulaFIT BURN™ is designed to help boost fat burning and provide a sense of wellbeing that reduces cravings for food and snacking.

When combined with a healthy diet and exercise, BURN capsules promote a sense of well being and energy that reduces cravings for food and snacking. BURN can also play an important role in increasing the results of ketosis and even avoiding the 'keto flu' that some people may experience with other ketogenic programs."

Huh? What's keto flu? I figured a site with the name Keto Size Me (http://ketosizeme.com/keto-flu-101-everything-need-know/) could help us out here... and they did. "The 'keto flu' is what we commonly call carbohydrate withdrawal symptoms. These symptoms usually occur in people who start a low carb diet that alters their hormones and causes and electrolyte imbalances."

Wait! Electrolyte imbalances? But we work so hard with the renal diet trying to keep these within the proper range for CKD. I went back to *What Is It and How Did I Get It? Early Stage Chronic Kidney Disease* for a little reminder about electrolytes.

"In order to fully understand the renal diet, you need to know a little something about electrolytes. There are the sodium, potassium, and phosphate you've been told about and also calcium, magnesium, chloride, and bicarbonate. They maintain balance in your body....Too much or too little of a certain electrolyte presents different problems."

4/24/17 *So That's How It's Decided*

***SlowItDownCKD*'s** being honored as one of the best kidney disease blogs for 2016 has had some interesting results. The first was the health and food writer's guest blog about hydration for Chronic Kidney Disease on March 6th. Then it was the guest blog by the Social Security Administration's Outreach Director. This week, it's a telephone interview with Dr. Michael J. Germain, a nephrologist from Massachusetts, about some of the suggested guidelines in the upcoming KDIGO for 2016.

Got it: backtrack. Let's start with KDIGO. This stands for KIDNEY DISEASE | IMPROVING GLOBAL OUTCOMES. Their homepage at KDIGO.org states,

"**KDIGO MISSION –** Improving the care and outcomes of kidney disease patients worldwide through the development and implementation of global clinical practice guidelines."

Anyone up for visiting their offices? What an excuse to go to Belgium!

Okay, now we know what the organization is and what it does, but why Dr. Germain? I asked the same question. Although he is not on the KDIGO panel of doctors who decide what the next year's development and implementation will be, he is well versed with the topic having published or having been part of the writing for an overwhelming number of articles in such esteemed journals as *the American Journal of Kidney Disease, Kidney International,* and *The Clinical Journal of the American Society of Nephrology,* as well as contributing to textbooks, … and he could simplify the medicalese in the guidelines to simple English for this lay person.

If you think I remind you quite often that I'm not a doctor, you should read my emails to our liaison. State I'm not a doctor, repeat, state I'm not a doctor, repeat. She had the good graces to laugh at my insecurities.

The latest guideline updates have not been released yet, so both the good doctor (over 40 years as a nephrologist) and I (CKD patient and awareness advocate for a decade) were working off the draft that was released last August

.

Dr. Germain also made it a point to ensure that I understand the guidelines are based upon expert opinion, not evidence. That made sense to me since he is not only a patient seeing nephrologist, but also a research nephrologist – to which his numerous publications will attest. With me being a lay person, he "had a lot of 'splaining to do." I had to admire his passion when discussing the vitamin D guidelines.

In the draft guidelines, it was suggested that hypercalcemia be avoided. I know; it's a new word. We already know that hyper is a prefix meaning over or too much; think excessive in this case. Calcemia looks sort of like calcium.

Good thinking because, according to Healthline at http://www.healthline.com/health/hypercalcemia:

"Hypercalcemia is a condition in which you have too high a concentration of calcium in your blood. Calcium performs important functions, such as helping keep your bones healthy. However, too much of it can cause problems...."

This excerpt from *What Is It and How Did I Get It? Early Stage Chronic Kidney Disease* explains how calcium works with vitamin D and phosphorous.

"The kidneys produce calcitrol which is the active form of vitamin D. The kidneys are the organs that transfer this vitamin from your food and skin [sunshine provides it to your skin] into something your body can use. Both vitamin D and calcium are needed for strong bones. It is yet another job of your kidneys to keep your bones strong and healthy. Should you have a deficit of Vitamin D, you'll need to be treated for this, in addition for any abnormal level of calcium or phosphates. The three work together. Vitamin D enables the calcium from the food you eat to be absorbed in the body. CKD may leech the calcium from your bones and body."

The Book of Blogs: Moderate Stage Chronic Kidney Disease, Part 2 offers us more information.

"The parathyroid glands are located in the neck, near or attached to the back side of the thyroid gland. Parathyroid hormone controls calcium, phosphorus, and vitamin D levels in the blood and bone. Release of PTH is controlled by the level of calcium in the blood. Low blood calcium levels cause increased PTH to be released, while high blood calcium levels block PTH release. ...

Thanks to MedLine Plus at http://www.nlm.nih.gov/medlineplus/ency/article/003690.htm ."

As Dr. Germain explained, CKD patients break down vitamin D quickly since they have more of a catabolic enzyme, the enzyme that converts the vitamin D to an inactive form. Oh, right, catabolic means "any destructive process by which complex substances are converted by living cells into more simple compounds, with release of energy" according to *Dorland's Medical Dictionary for Health Consumers*.

Here's the problem: vitamin D can cause hypercalcemia. Dr. Germain phrased it, "In fact, the draft guideline recommends active vitamin D hormone therapy not to be routinely used in patients with CKD stage 3 or 4 due to increased risk of hypercalcemia and the lack of efficacy shown in studies." Therefore, he urges nephrologists to wait until stage 4 or 5 to recommend vitamin D since hyperparathyroidism *may* lead to bone damage. But just as in any disease, it is harder to treat bone damage once it's already there. His recommendation: Ask about your parathyroid level every three to six months and discuss the results of your tests with your nephrologist. By the way, his feeling – and obviously mine – is that preserving the kidney function is the most important job of the nephrologist and the patient.

I am eager to see the guidelines published so I can write more about them. The conclusion about vitamin D is based upon what nephrologists have seen in their practices since the last set of KDIGO guidelines were published in 2009. It will affect the way our nephrologists speak with us about our treatment, just as the other guidelines for 2016 will.

That will affect the way we self-manage. For example, I restrict my sun time to 15 minutes a day based on these findings. Take a look at how you self-manage. It should bring up a list of questions for you to ask your nephrologist at your next appointment.

You should also know the KDIGO deals with all stages of CKD including End Stage CKD and pediatric CKD.

5/1/17 *Getting a Little Too High*

You know those blood and urine tests you take periodically? Have you ever looked at your uric acid levels? It might be worth the effort. This is from **What Is It and How Did I Get It? Early Stage Chronic Kidney Disease**:

"Uric Acid levels in the blood can indicate that you're at risk for gout, kidney stones, or kidney failure. It's the kidney's job to filter uric acid from the body. A buildup means the kidneys are not doing their job well."

For the first time ever – and I've had Chronic Kidney Disease for nine years – my uric acid levels were high. Why now? What could this mean? I already know I have Chronic Kidney Disease. I haven't had a kidney stone in nine years and was unaware of having that one until my nephrologist told me I did. Is it gout?

Time to back track. What is uric acid anyway?

In **The Book of Blogs: Moderate Stage Chronic Kidney Disease, Part 2** (Hang on; I'm working on simplifying that title.), I used the Merriam Webster Dictionary at https://www.merriam-webster.com/dictionary/uric%20acid for this definition:

"**URIC ACID**: a white odorless and tasteless nearly insoluble acid $C_5H_4N_4O_3$ that is the chief nitrogenous waste present in the urine especially of lower vertebrates (as birds and reptiles), is present in small quantity in human urine, and occurs pathologically in renal calculi {A little help here: this means a concretion usually of mineral salts around organic material found especially in hollow organs or ducts} and the tophi of gout."

Back to gout, in **SlowItDownCKD 2016**, I wrote a little bit about one of the causes of gout: purines in our diet.

"According to WebMD
at http://www.webmd.com/arthritis/tc/diet-and-gout-topic-overview:

'Purines (specific chemical compounds found in some foods) are broken down into uric acid. A diet rich in purines from certain sources can raise uric acid levels in the body, which sometimes leads to gout. Meat and seafood may increase your risk of gout. Dairy products may lower your risk.'

It seems to me a small list of high purine foods is appropriate here. Gout Education at http://gouteducation.org/patient/gout-treatment/diet/ offers just that. This also appears to be an extremely helpful site for those wanting to know more about gout. "Because uric acid is formed from the breakdown of purines, high-purine foods can trigger attacks. It is strongly encouraged to avoid:

- Beer and grain liquors
- Red meat, lamb and pork
- Organ meats, such as liver, kidneys and sweetbreads
- Seafood, especially shellfish, like shrimp, lobster, mussels, anchovies and sardines"

This doesn't work for me. Except for shrimp which I'll have two or three times a year, I don't eat or drink any of this food. Grrrrr. Back to the drawing board. Let me see if I can find other causes of high uric acid levels. The Mayo Clinic at http://www.mayoclinic.org/symptoms/high-uric-acid-level/basics/causes/sym-20050607 had some other suggestions:

"Factors that may cause a high uric acid level in your blood include:
- Diuretic medications (water pills)
- Drinking too much alcohol
- Genetics (inherited tendencies)

- Hypothyroidism(underactive thyroid)
- Immune-suppressing drugs
- Niacin, or vitamin B-3
- Obesity
- Psoriasis
- Purine-rich diet — liver, game meat, anchovies, sardines, gravy, dried beans and peas, mushrooms, and other foods
- Renal insufficiency — inability of the kidneys to filter waste
- Tumor lysis syndrome — a rapid release of cells into the blood caused by certain cancers or by chemotherapy for those cancers

Also, you may be monitored for high uric acid levels when undergoing chemotherapy or radiation treatment for cancer."

As far as I know, I don't have an inherited tendency toward high uric acid levels. Nor do I have hypothyroidism, take immune-suppressing drugs, niacin, or vitamin B-3. We already know that I don't drink alcohol or eat purine rich foods, and have CKD. I've never been treated for cancer, so what's left?

Hmmm, I do take a diuretic, am obese, and have psoriasis. Wait a minute. I thought diuretics helped you reduce the amount of water and salt in your body. Now they may cause high uric acid? How? Drugs.com at https://www.drugs.com/health-guide/gout.html helped me out here:

"The kidneys do not excrete enough uric acid. This can be caused by kidney disease, starvation and alcohol use, especially binge drinking. This also can occur in people taking medications called diuretics (such as hydrochlorothiazide or furosemide)."

Time to speak with my doctor about this prescription, I think.

My psoriasis is so latent that I often forget I have it. However, Arthritis.org at http://www.arthritis.org/about-arthritis/types/psoriatic-arthritis/articles/psoriatic-arthritis-increases-gout-risk.php tells us:

"In gout, uric acid builds up in the joints and tissue around the joints – often the big toe – and forms needle-like crystals, which can cause sudden episodes of intense pain and swelling. If left untreated, gout can become chronic and lead to joint damage. In psoriasis and psoriatic arthritis, uric acid is thought to be a by-product of rapid skin cell turnover and systemic inflammation."

That also explains what gout is, which I'd neglected to do. Something kept nagging at my memory (oh, to have a clear memory without the nagging for a change.) Got it. It was in *SlowItDown 2016*:

"Ah, we know Chronic Kidney Disease is an inflammatory disease. Now we know that arthritis is, too. Being a purist over here, I wanted to check on psoriasis to see if falls into this category, too. Oh my! According to a Position Statement from the American Academy of Dermatologists and AAD Association:

'Psoriasis is a chronic inflammatory, multi-system disease associated with considerable morbidity and co-morbid conditions.'

Arthritis is an inflammatory disease; psoriasis is an inflammatory disease; and Chronic Kidney Disease is an inflammatory disease. The common factor here is obvious – inflammatory disease."

I'm beginning to see the pattern here. Well, what about the weight? I discovered this quote on The Arthritis Foundation's Gout Blog at http://blog.arthritis.org/gout/weight-gout-risk/ :

"'Higher weight is associated with higher uric acid levels in the blood, which therefore increases gout risk,' says Tuhina Neogi, MD, PhD, associate professor of medicine at Boston University School of Medicine."

That strong connection between inflammation and weight leaves me speechless. It seems so transparent, yet I somehow manage to forget it repeatedly. Ugh!

5/8/17 *Recreating Creatinine*

I throw a lot of terms around as if we all understood them. Sorry for that. One reader made it clear he needed more information about creatinine. In another part of my life, I belong to a community that calls reviewing or further explanation of a certain topic recreating… and today I'm going to recreate creatinine.

Let's start in the beginning. This is what I wrote in the beginning of my CKD awareness advocacy in **What Is It and How Did I Get It? Early Stage Chronic Kidney Disease** :

"Creatinine is a waste product of muscle activity. What actually happens is that our bodies use protein to build muscles and repair themselves. This used protein becomes an amino acid which enters the blood and ends up in the liver where it is once again changed. This time it's changed into urea which goes through the kidneys into the urine.

The harder the muscles work, the more creatinine that is produced and carried by the blood to the kidneys where it also enters the urine. This in itself is not toxic, but measuring the urea and creatinine shows the level of the clearance of the harmful toxins the body does produce. These harmful toxins do build up if not voided until a certain level is reached which can make us ill. Working kidneys filter this creatinine from your blood. When the blood levels of creatinine rise, you know your kidneys are slowing down. During my research, I discovered that a non-CKD patient's blood is cleaned about 35 times a day. A CKD patient's blood is cleaned progressively fewer times a day depending upon the stage of the patient's disease."

Got it. Well, I did have to read it a couple of times to get it straight in my mind. Now what? Let's see what more information I can find about what this means to a CKD patient. **The Book of Blogs: Mod-**

erate Stage Chronic Kidney Disease, Part 1 contains the following explanation from DaVita,

"Because there are often no symptoms of kidney disease, laboratory tests are critical. When you get a screening, a trained technician will draw blood that will be tested for creatinine, a waste product. If kidney function is abnormal, creatinine levels will increase in the blood, due to decreased excretion of creatinine in the urine. Your glomerular filtration rate (GFR) will then be calculated, which factors in age, gender, creatinine and ethnicity. The GFR indicates the person's stage of Chronic Kidney Disease which provides an evaluation of kidney function."

I thought you might want to know more about this test, so I turned to *The Book of Blogs: Moderate Stage Chronic Kidney Disease, Part 2* since I remembered including The National Kidney Disease Education Program at The U.S. Department of Health and Human Services' information (including some reminders about definitions) concerning the process of being tested for CKD.

1. "A blood test checks your GFR, which tells how well your kidneys are filtering....
2. A urine test checks for albumin. Albumin is a protein that can pass into the urine when the kidneys are damaged.
3.

If necessary, meaning if your kidney function is compromised, your PCP will make certain you get to a nephrologist promptly. This specialist will conduct more intensive tests that include:

Blood:
BUN – BUN stands for blood urea nitrogen.
Creatinine – The creatinine blood test measures the level of creatinine in the blood. This test is done to see how well your kidneys work.

Urine:
Creatinine clearance – The creatinine clearance test helps provide information about how well the kidneys are working. The test compares the creatinine level in urine with the creatinine level in blood."

Aha! So there are two different creatinine readings: blood or serum and urine. By the way, MedicineNet at http://www.medicinenet.com/script/main/art.asp?articlekey=5470 defines serum as

"The clear liquid that can be separated from clotted blood. Serum differs from plasma, the liquid portion of normal unclotted blood containing the red and white cells and platelets. It is the clot that makes the difference between serum and plasma."

This is starting to get pretty complex. It seems that yet another test for CKD can be conducted with a urine sample. This is from *SlowItDownCKD 2015*.

"In recent years, researchers have found that a single urine sample can provide the needed information. In the newer technique, the amount of albumin in the urine sample is compared with the amount of creatinine, a waste product of normal muscle breakdown. The measurement is called a urine albumin-to-creatinine ratio (UACR). A urine sample containing more than 30 milligrams of albumin for each gram of creatinine (30 mg/g) is a warning that there may be a problem. If the laboratory test exceeds 30 mg/g, another UACR test should be done 1 to 2 weeks later. If the second test also shows high levels of protein, the person has persistent proteinuria, a sign of declining kidney function, and should have additional tests to evaluate kidney function.

Thank you to the National Kidney and Urologic Diseases Information Clearinghouse, A service of the NIH, at http://kidney.niddk.nih.gov/kudiseases/pubs/proteinuria/#tests for that information."

Is there more to know about creatinine? Uh-oh, this savory little tidbit was reprinted in *SlowItDownCKD 2016* from an earlier book.

"....Dr. HL Trivedi of the Institute of Kidney Diseases and Research Centre (IKDRC) said, '…. Rapid water loss causes the kidney's functioning to slow down, resulting in temporary or permanent kidney failure.'

Extreme heat causes rapid water loss, resulting in acute electrolyte imbalance. The kidney, unable to cope with the water loss, fails to flush out the requisite amount of Creatinine and other toxins from the body. Coupled with a lack of consistent water intake, this brings about permanent or temporary kidney failure, explain experts."

This seems to be calling for a Part 2. What do you think? There's still BUN and albumin to deal with. Let me know what else you'd like to see included in that blog.

5/15/17 B.U.N. No, not bun. B.U.N.

Let's consider this part 2 of last week's blog since all these terms and tests and functions are intertwined for Chronic Kidney Disease patients. Thanks to reader Paul (not my Bear, but another Paul) for emphatically agreeing with me about this.

Bing! Bing! Bing! I know where to start. This is from The National Kidney Disease Education Program at the U.S. Department of Health and Human Services' information about being tested for CKD.

"If necessary, meaning if your kidney function is compromised, your pcp will make certain you get to a nephrologist promptly. This specialist will conduct more intensive tests that include:

Blood:
BUN –
BUN stands for blood urea nitrogen. Urea nitrogen is what forms when protein breaks down."

If you read last week's blog about creatinine, you know there's more to the testing than that and that more of the information is in *The Book of Blogs: Moderate Stage Chronic Kidney Disease, Part 2*. No sense to repeat myself so soon.

Let's take this very slowly. I don't think it necessary to define blood, but urea? Maybe. I found this in *SlowItDownCKD 2015*:

"But how can I explain blood urea? I'll allow the experts to do that.
http://www.patient.co.uk/health/routine-kidney-function-blood-test has the simplest explanation.

'Urea is a waste product formed from the breakdown of proteins. Urea is usually passed out in the urine. A high blood level of urea ('uraemia') indicates that the kidneys may not be working properly or that you are dehydrated (have low body water content).'

In the U.S., we call this test B.U.N. or Blood Urea Nitrogen Blood Test. So as I understand it, if your protein intake is high, more urea is produced. But since your kidneys are already compromised by CKD, the toxins remaining in your body are not eliminated as well...."

You with me so far? If there's suspicion of CKD, your nephrologist tests your serum creatinine (see last week's blog) and your BUN. Wait a minute; I haven't explained nitrogen yet. Oh, I see; it has to be defined in conjunction with urea.

Thanks to The National Kidney Foundation at https://www.kidney.org/atoz/content/understanding-your-lab-values for clearing this up:

"Urea nitrogen is a normal waste product in your blood that comes from the breakdown of protein from the foods you eat and from your body metabolism. It is normally removed from your blood by your kidneys, but when kidney function slows down, the BUN level rises. BUN can also rise if you eat more protein, and it can fall if you eat less protein."

So now the reason for this protein restriction I wrote about in **What Is It and How Did I Get It? Early Stage Chronic Kidney Disease** should be clear.

"So, why is protein limited? One reason is that it is the source of a great deal of phosphorus. Another is that a number of nephrons were already destroyed before you were even diagnosed. Logically, those that remain compensate for those that are no longer viable. The remaining nephrons are doing more work than they were meant to. Just like a car that is pushed too hard, there will be constant deterioration if you don't stop pushing. The idea is to stop pushing your remaining nephrons to work even harder in an attempt to slow down the advancement of your CKD. Restricting protein is a way to reduce the nephrons' work."

This is starting to sound like a rabbit warren – one piece leads to another, which verves off to lead to another, and so forth and so on. All right, let's keep going anyway.

Guess what. Urea is also tested via the urine. Nothing like confusing the issue, at least to those of us who are lay people like me. Let's see if Healthline at http://www.healthline.com/health/urea-nitrogen-urine#overview1 can straighten this out for us.

"Your body creates ammonia when it breaks down protein from foods. Ammonia contains nitrogen, which mixes with other elements in your body, including carbon, hydrogen, and oxygen to form urea. Urea is a waste product that is excreted by the kidneys when you urinate.

The urine urea nitrogen test determines how much urea is in the urine to assess the amount of protein breakdown. The test can help determine how well the kidneys are functioning, and if your intake of protein is too high or low. Additionally, it can help diagnose whether you have a problem with protein digestion or absorption from the gut."

Hmmm, these two don't sound that different to me other than what is being analyzed for the result – blood (although blood serum is used, rather than whole blood) or urine.

What about BUN to Creatinine tests? How do they fit in here? After all, this is part 2 of last week's blog about creatinine. Thank

you to Medicine Net at
http://www.medicinenet.com/creatinine_blood_test/article.htm
for explaining.

"The BUN-to-creatinine ratio generally provides more precise information about kidney function and its possible underlying cause
compared with creatinine level alone."

Dizzy yet? I think that's enough for one day.

Did you know you can loan my books to a Kindle friend or borrow
them from one for free for 14 days? Or you can ask your local li-
brarian to order them, another way of reading them free. I almost
forgot: if you are a member of Kindle Unlimited and the Kindle
Owners' Lending Library, you can read the books for free (although you do need to pay your usual monthly subscription fee).
Students: Please be aware that some unscrupulous sites have
been offering to rent you my books for a term for much more than
it would cost to buy them. I've succeeded in getting most of them
to stop this practice, but more keep popping up.

5/22/17 *Ratio: Is That Like Rationing?*

A friend called me Friday night wondering what her creatinine/albumin ratio meant since that reading was high on her last blood draw. Actually, she wanted to know if this was something to worry about. After extracting a promise that she would call her doctor with her questions today when her physician's office opened for business again, I gave her some explanations. Of course, then I wanted to give you the same explanations.

Although the Online Etymology Dictionary tells us both ratio and rationing are derived from the same Latin root – *ratio* – which means

"reckoning, calculation; business affair, procedure," also "reason, reasoning, judgment, understanding,"

they aren't exactly the same. My old favorite, The Merriam-Webster Dictionary defines ratio at https://www.merriam-webster.com/dictionary/ratio in the following way:

"the relationship in quantity, amount, or size between two or more things"

as in that of your creatinine and albumin.

As for rationing, if you're old enough to remember World War II, you know what it means. If you're not, the same dictionary can help us out again. At https://www.merriam-webster.com/dictionary/rationing, we're told it's "a share especially as determined by supply."

Nope, doesn't work here since we're not sharing our creatinine or albumin with anyone else. We each have our own supply in our own ratios, albeit sometimes too high or sometimes too low.

What are creatinine and albumin anyway? Let's see what we can find about creatinine in *What Is It and How Did I Get It? Early Stage Chronic Kidney Disease.*

"Additional important jobs of the kidneys are removing liquid waste from your body and balancing the minerals in the body. The two liquid waste products are urea which has been broken down from protein by the digestive system and creatinine which is a by-product of muscle activity."

Well, what about albumin? This can get a bit complicated. Remember, the UACR (Hang on, explanation of this coming soon.) deals with urine albumin. There's an explanation in *SlowItDownCKD 2016* about what it's not: serum albumin.

"Maybe we should take a look at serum albumin level. Serum means it's the clear part of your blood, the part without red or white blood cells. This much is fairly common knowledge. Albumin is not. MedlinePlus, part of The National Institutes of Health's U.S. National Library of Medicine at https://medlineplus.gov/ency/article/003480.htm tells us,

'Albumin is a protein made by the liver. A serum albumin test measures the amount of this protein in the clear liquid portion of the blood.'

Uh-oh, this is also not good: a high level of serum albumin indicates progression of your kidney disease. Conversely, kidney disease can cause a high level of serum albumin."

This is from *SlowItDownCKD 2015* and explains what the UACR is and why your albumin-to-creatinine ratio (UAC R) is important:

"In recent years, researchers have found that a single urine sample can provide the needed information. In the newer technique, the amount of albumin in the urine sample is compared with the amount of creatinine, a waste product of normal muscle breakdown. The measurement is called a urine albumin-to-creatinine ratio (UACR). A urine sample containing more than 30 milligrams of albumin for each gram of creatinine (30 mg/g) is a warning that there may be a problem. If the laboratory test exceeds 30 mg/g, another UACR test should be done 1 to 2 weeks later. If the second test also shows high levels of protein, the person has persistent proteinuria, a sign of declining kidney function, and should have additional tests to evaluate kidney function.

Thank you to the National Kidney and Urologic Diseases Information Clearinghouse , a service of the NIH, at http://kidney.niddk.nih.gov/kudiseases/pubs/proteinuria/#tests for that information."

Basically, that means if you have a high UACR once, get your urine retested a week or two later before you even think about worrying, which is what my friend's doctor confirmed. But do make sure to get that second test so you can be certain your kidney function is not being compromised.

I was thrilled that both my paper and notes from the field about Chronic Kidney Disease Awareness were accepted for Landmark's Journal for the Conference for Global Transformation AND then be able to present a poster about it during the conference this past weekend. In addition I was lucky enough to have lunch with one of the keynote speakers.

Who, you ask? Amy D. Waterman, Ph.D. This is one important person to us. She has changed the face of pre dialysis and transplant education globally by starting "an educational nonprofit corporation and has been awarded more than $20 million in grants...she has reached tens of thousands of people to date, educating them in the miracle of live organ donation. Last year, Dr.

Waterman was invited to the White House to share about the possibility of ending the organ donor shortage." This material is from the *Journal of the 2017 Conference for Global Transformation, Volume 17, No. 1.*

This is exactly what we need to do for early and moderate stage CKD. This is what the social media presence, the blogs, and the books are about. And you know what? That's just.plain.not.enough. Last I heard, I have 107,000 readers in 106 countries. And you know what? That's just.plain.not.enough. Am I greedy? Absolutely when it comes to sharing awareness of CKD. Do I know how to expand my coverage? Nope...not yet, that is. I am so very open to suggestions? Let me hear them!

5/29/17 CKD and the VA or It's Not Alphabet Soup at All

Today is Memorial Day in the United States. It is not a day to say Happy Memorial Day since it is a day commemorating those who gave their lives for our freedom. Lots of us have bar-b-ques or go to the park or the beach to celebrate. No problem there as long as we remember WHO we are celebrating. I promise: no political rant here, just plain appreciation of those who serve(d) us both living and dead. Personally, I am honoring my husband, my step son-in-law, and all those cousins who just never came home again. I explained the origins of this day in *SlowItDownCKD 2015*, so won't re-explain it here. You can go to the blog and just scroll down to that month and year in the drop down menu on the right side of the page under Archives or you can look at the blog entry for May 25th in the book.

We already know that Chronic Kidney Disease will prevent you from serving your country in the military, although there are so many other ways to serve our country. This is from *The Book of Blogs: Moderate Stage Chronic Kidney Disease, Part 2*:

'The Department of Defense's Instruction for Medical Standards for Appointment, Enlistment, or Induction in the Military Services establishes medical standards, which, if not met, are grounds for rejection for military service. Other standards may be prescribed for a mobilization for a national emergency.

As of September 13, 2011, according to Change 1 of this Instruction, the following was included.

'Current or history of acute (580) nephritis or chronic (582) Chronic Kidney Disease of any type.'

Until this date, Chronic Kidney Disease was not mentioned."

You can read the entire list of The Department of Defense's Instruction for Medical Standards for Appointment, Enlistment, or Induction in the Military Services at http://dtic.mil/whs/directives/corres/pdf/613003p.pdf. You'll also find information there about metabolic syndrome, high blood pressure, high cholesterol, diabetes, and pre-diabetes as conditions for non-enlistment.

This got me to thinking. What if you were had already enlisted when you developed CKD. Yes, you would be discharged as medically unfit, but could you get help as a veteran?

According to the Veterans Administration at https://www.research.va.gov/topics/Kidney_disease.cfm#research4,

"In 2012, VA and the University of Michigan began the work of creating a national kidney disease registry to monitor kidney disease among Veterans. The registry will provide accurate and timely information about the burden and trends related to kidney disease among Veterans and identify Veterans at risk for kidney disease.

VA hopes the kidney disease registry will lead to improvements in access to care, such as kidney transplants. The department also expects the registry will allow VA clinicians to better monitor and prevent kidney disease, and will reduce costs related to kidney disease."

That's what was hoped for five years ago. Let's see if it really came to fruition.

Oh, this is promising and taken directly from The U.S. Department of Veterans Affairs.

"VA eKidney Clinic

The VA eKidney Clinic is now available! The eKidney Clinic offers patient education through interactive virtual classrooms where Veterans can learn how to take care of their kidneys and live a good life with kidney disease. Please visit the VA eKidney Clinic website or click on the picture below. For additional information see the eKidney Clinic Patient Information Brochure."

The Veterans Health Administration doesn't just provide information, although I must say I was delighted to see the offer of Social Work Services. There is also treatment available. Notice dialysis mentioned in their mission statement.

"**Mission:** The VHA Kidney Program's mission is to improve the quality and consistency of healthcare services delivered to Veterans with kidney disease nationwide. The VHA Kidney Program provides kidney-related services to dialysis centers throughout VA's medical centers. Professional guidance and services are available in the form of consultation and policies developed by VA kidney experts. These experts are dedicated to furthering the understanding of kidney disease, its impact on Veterans, and developing treatments to help patients manage disease symptoms. In addition, the VHA Kidney Program provides VA healthcare professionals with clinical care, education, research, and informatics resources to improve healthcare at local VA dialysis facilities."

I did find it strange that there was a cravat on the Veterans Administration site that they do not necessarily endorse the VHA Kidney Program, especially since it is so helpful.

How involved is the VA with CKD patients? These are the 2015 statistics:
- All Veterans enrolled in VA are eligible for services, regardless of service connection status

- Enrolled Veterans can receive services from the VA or from community providers under the Non-VA Care Program if VA services are unavailable
- 49 VA health care facilities offer kidney disease specialty care (nephrology services)
- 96 VA facilities offer inpatient and/or outpatient dialysis; 25 centers are inpatient-only. Of the 71 VA outpatient dialysis centers, 64 are hospital based units, 2 are joint VA/DoD units, 4 are freestanding units, and one is within a community based outpatient clinic (CBOC)
- VA enrollees must be offered the option of home dialysis provided either directly by the VA or through the Non-VA Care Program
- 36 outpatient hemodialysis centers offer home dialysis care directly.
- 5 VA medical centers host kidney transplantation programs.
- VA Delivered Kidney Care (Calendar Year 2013) 13,794 Unique Veterans receiving dialysis paid for by VA; representing an annual increase of 13% since 2008. 794 Veterans received home dialysis; 55percent (434) by VA facilities and 45percent (360) under the Non-VA Care Program.
- Increasing use of telehealth services to increase Veteran access to kidney specialty care Secure messaging: 7,319 messages, Clinical video telehealth: 4,977 encounters
- VA Kidney Research (FY '14) the research budget for the study of kidney disease has been $18.5 million per year for the past 5 years (FY '10-FY '14). The VA Cooperative Studies Program has supported national clinical trials addressing the best treatment of Veterans with CKD since at least 1998.

It seems to me our veterans are covered. Now if we could only make sure the rest of us stay covered no matter what bills the current administration signs into law.

6/5/17 *How Did It Get Political?*

A couple of weeks ago, I wrote about Dr. Amy D. Waterman at UCLA's Division of Nephrology's Transplant Research and Education Center. We'd met at Landmark's 2017 Conference for Global Transformation. She has brought to the world of dialysis and transplant the kind of education I want to see offered for Chronic Kidney Disease. I also asked for ideas as to how I could help in developing this kind of contribution to CKD awareness… and the universe answered.

First the bad news, so you can tell when the good news come in. Here in the U.S., The *National Kidney Foundation* at https://www.kidney.org/news/national-kidney-foundation-statement-macarthur-amendment-to-american-health-care-act issued the following statement on May 3 of this year:

"The National Kidney Foundation opposes the American Health Care Act (AHCA) as amended. The amendment to AHCA, offered by Representative Tom MacArthur (R-NJ), raises significant concerns for millions of Americans affected by chronic diseases. If this bill passes, National Kidney Foundation is highly concerned that insurers in some states will be granted additional flexibility to charge higher premiums, and apply annual and lifetime limits on benefits without a limit on out-of-pocket costs for those with pre-existing conditions, including chronic kidney disease. The bill also permits waivers on Federal protections regarding essential health benefits which could limit patient access to the medications and care they need to manage their conditions. These limits could also include access to dialysis and transplantation. For these reasons, we must oppose the legislation as amended.

In addition, National Kidney Foundation is concerned that the elimination of income based tax credits and cost sharing subsidies, combined with the reduction in funds to Medicaid, will reduce the number of people who will obtain coverage; many of whom have, or are at risk for, chronic kidney disease (CKD)."

The world sees what stress Trump is causing our country (as well as our planet.) Yet, there is hope in the form of a new bill. "... the bill — introduced in the House by Reps. Tom Marino (R-Pennsylvania), John Lewis (D-Georgia) and Peter Roskam (R-Illinois) — aims to:

• Have the Department of Health and Human Services (HHS) and U.S. Government Accountability Office (GAO) issue a series of recommendations to Congress on "how to increase kidney transplantation rates; how palliative care can be used to improve the quality of life for those living with kidney disease; and how to better understand kidney disease in minority populations" – to back federal research efforts;
• Create an economically sustainable dialysis infrastructure and modernized quality programs to improve patient care and quality outcomes — for instance, by creating incentives to work in poorer communities and rural areas;
• Increase access to treatment and managed care for patients with a confirmed diagnosis of kidney disease by ensuring Medigap coverage for people living with ESRD, promoting access to home dialysis and allow patients with ESRD to keep their private insurance coverage.

According to the National Kidney Foundation, more than 660,000 Americans are receiving treatment for ESRD. Of these, 468,000 are undergoing dialysis and more than 193,000 have a functioning kidney transplant."

Thank you to the CDC at https://ckdnews.com/2017/05/31/ckd-end-stage-renal-disease-patients-benefit-bipartisan-bill-kidney-care-partners/ for this encouraging news. Although it's just a newly introduced bill at this time, notice the educational aspects of the first point.

For those outside the U.S, who may not know what it is, this is how Medicare was defined in *What Is It and How Did I Get It? Early Stage Chronic Kidney Disease*

"U.S. government health insurance for those over 65, those having certain special needs, or those who have end stage renal disease."

An interview with Trump while he was campaigning last year was included in *SlowItDownCKD 2016*, (11/14/16) This is what he had to say about medical coverage for those of us with pre-existing conditions like CKD. (Lesley Stahl is the well-respected interviewer.)

"Lesley Stahl: Let me ask you about Obamacare (Me here: that's our existing health care coverage.), which you say you're going to repeal and replace. When you replace it, are you going to make sure that people with pre-conditions are still covered?

Donald Trump: Yes. Because it happens to be one of the strongest assets.' ....

What does the president elect say about Medicare? Those of us over 65 (That's me.) have Medicare as our primary insurance. I am lucky enough to have a secondary insurance through my union. How many of the rest of us are? By the way, if Medicare doesn't' pay, neither does my secondary."

This is from the same book:

"Here's what Trump had to say in a rally in Iowa on December 11th of last year (e.g. meaning 2015).

'So, you've been paying into Social Security and Medicare…but we are not going to cut your Social Security and we're not cutting your Medicare….'"

We do not have the most truthful president here in the U.S., so you can see how even the introduction of the Marino, Lewis, Roskam bill is good news for us. While this is not meant to be a political blog, our pre-existing illness – our CKD – has caused many of us to unwittingly become political.

On another topic, a reader asked what the AAKP is. Their Mission Statement at https://aakp.org/mission/ tells us:

"The American Association of Kidney Patients is dedicated to improving the quality of life for kidney patients through education, advocacy, patient engagement and the fostering of patient communities.

Education
The American Association of Kidney Patients (AAKP) is recognized as the leader for patient-centered education – continually developing high quality, professionally written, edited and reviewed educational pieces covering every level of kidney disease.
Advocacy
For more than 40 years, AAKP has been the patient voice – advocating for improved access to high-quality health care through regulatory and legislative reform at the federal level. The Association's work has improved long term outcomes in both quality of health and the ability for patients and family members affected by kidney disease to lead a more productive and meaningful life.
Community
AAKP is leading the effort to bring kidney patients together to promote community, conversations and to seek out services that help maximize patients' everyday lives."

6/12/17   *Here, There, and Everywhere*

AAKP is the acronym for the American Association of Kidney Patients. I am flabbergasted that six patients in Brooklyn, New York, started this group in 1969 while they were undergoing dialysis and that today AAKP reaches one million people at all stages of kidney disease. I'm a member as of last week. Did I mention that membership is free?

Before I start to sound like I'm selling you a product, here's their web site so you can explore this association for yourself: https://aakp.org.

Let's say you don't want to travel. How else can you partake of the kidney patient world, the part of it that doesn't deal with going to the nephrologist or renal dietician? Well, have you heard of Renal Support Network at http://www.rsnhope.org/? Lori Hartwell has had kidney disease since she was two years old and wanted to instill hope in those with the disease. Now you understand the URL. There are also podcasts about kidney disease at http://www.rsnhope.org/kidneytalk-podcast/ or you can go through the menu on their home page.

Lori was especially helpful to me when I was first starting out in CKD awareness advocacy. I think you'll find something of interest to you on her website, although I'll bet it won't be the same something for any two people. What I especially like is the Health Library with articles on varied subjects.

Further afield, The Bhutan Kidney Foundation is doing an Amazonian job of spreading kidney disease awareness. I am constantly reading about their walks and educational meetings, as well as governmental initiatives. I think they may even have a Facebook page. Let me go check. Hi again. I'm back and they do.

Have you heard of Mani Trust? This is an India based group that strives to provide humanitarian help to individuals and their country, including those suffering from kidney disease. We know this is not a Western-part-of-the-world-only problem, but I wonder if we realize just how widespread it is.

Remember I told you about the CKD awareness presentation I offered at a global conference several weeks ago? I found astounding facts from World Life Expectancy at http://www.worldlifeexpectancy.com. One of the most striking facts I included in that presentation is that globally 864,226 people died of kidney disease last year. That makes kidney disease number 15 in the cause of death hit parade.

In Malaysia, there were 2,768 deaths due to kidney disease, over 2% of the country's total population. In Albania, there were 443; that's also close to 2% of the country's total population. Ghana had 2,469 deaths, which is 1.3%. Egypt? 15,820, which is almost 3½ %. Here in the United States, there were 59,186 deaths, which is almost 3% of our population. What's my point?

Kidney disease is a global problem. I don't know what I can do to help in other countries in other parts of the world, but I do know what I can do to help here… and what you can do to help here. If you're able to, attend the national meetings and local conferences about kidney disease and spread whatever new information you've learned. If you are unable to travel, keep your eye on the Facebook kidney disease pages which often have files and delve into them. Share this information, too. If you don't travel and you're not on a computer, register for mailing lists and share information from them, too. Of course, check everything you read with your nephrologist before you share and use the advice yourself.

You'll find a blog roll – a list of kidney care and awareness organizations – on the right side of my blog. Why not explore some of these and see which ones appeal to you? If you like them, you'll read them. And, hopefully, if you read them, you'll share the information. According to the latest CDC findings, more than one out of every seven people in the United States has CKD. Let's try to change those figures.

6/19/17 *The Other Side of the Coin*

Here's hoping everyone had a wonderful Father's Day. During our relaxed celebration for Bear, I found myself ruminating about how many times we've celebrated this holiday for fathers no longer with us and how many more times we would be able to celebrate it for the fathers who are. They are aging. Wait a minute, that means their kidneys are aging, too.

Yep, that meant a new blog topic. We already know that kidney function declines with age. According to the National Kidney Foundation at https://www.kidney.org/blog/ask-doctor/what-age-do-kidneys-decline-function, "The general 'Rule of Thumb' is that kidney function begins to decline at age 40 and declines at a rate of about 1% per year beyond age forty. Rates may differ in different individuals." 40?

Well, what is a perfect kidney function score… if such exists? Back to the NKF, although they call this a 'normal' not 'perfect' GFR, this time at https://www.kidney.org/atoz/content/gfr:
In adults, the normal GFR number is more than 90. GFR declines with age, even in people without kidney disease.

Average estimated GFR

20–29	116
30–39	107
40–49	99
50–59	93
60–69	85
70+	75

Got it. So even for a normal 70+ person, I have CKD with my 50ish GFR.

It seems I'm getting a bit ahead of myself here. I haven't defined GFR yet. Let's take a gander at *What Is It and How Did I Get It? Early Stage Chronic Kidney Disease* for that definition,

"Glomerular filtration rate [if there is a lower case "e" before the term, it means estimated glomerular filtration rate] which determines both the stage of kidney disease and how well the kidneys are functioning."

No, that won't do. I think we need more of an explanation. This is from *SlowItDownCKD 2015*:

"Glomerular filtration rate (GFR) is a test used to check how well the kidneys are working. Specifically, it estimates how much blood passes through the glomeruli each minute. Glomeruli are the tiny filters in the kidneys that filter waste from the blood.

Many thanks to MedlinePlus at http://www.nlm.nih.gov/medlineplus/ency/article/007305.htm fo r the definition."

Okay, I think that's clear now. However, that's not what I wanted to know. This is – if kidney function already declines with age, does having CKD age us more quickly?

"**Premature aging** is a process associated with a progressive accumulation of deleterious changes over time, an impairment of physiologic functions, and an increase in the risk of disease and death. Regardless of genetic background, aging can be accelerated by the lifestyle choices and environmental conditions to which our genes are exposed. Chronic kidney disease is a common condition that promotes cellular senescence and premature aging through toxic alterations in the internal milieu. This occurs through several mechanisms, including DNA and mitochondria damage, increased reactive oxygen species generation, persistent inflammation, stem cell exhaustion, phosphate toxicity, decreased klotho expression, and telomere attrition...."

You can read the entire fascinating (to my way of thinking) in the *American Journal of Kidney Disease.*

Nature.com at http://www.nature.com/nrneph/journal/v10/n12/full/nrneph.2014.185.html seems to agree that CKD accelerates aging:

"Chronic kidney disease (CKD) shares many phenotypic similarities with other chronic diseases, including heart failure, chronic obstructive pulmonary disease, HIV infection and rheumatoid arthritis. The most apparent similarity is premature ageing, involving accelerated vascular disease and muscle wasting. We propose that in addition to a sedentary lifestyle and psychosocial and socioeconomic determinants, four major disease-induced mechanisms underlie premature ageing in CKD: an increase in allostatic load, activation of the 'stress resistance response', activation of age-promoting mechanisms and impairment of anti-ageing pathways.

The most effective current interventions to modulate premature ageing—treatment of the underlying disease, optimal nutrition, correction of the internal environment and exercise training—reduce systemic inflammation and oxidative stress and induce muscle anabolism. Deeper mechanistic insight into the phenomena of premature ageing as well as early diagnosis of CKD might improve the application and efficacy of these interventions and provide novel leads to combat muscle wasting and vascular impairment in chronic diseases."

Remember the friend of my daughters who hadn't seen me in five years who (thought) he whispered to her, "Your mom got so old." Now I understand why, although I have noticed this myself. I look in the mirror and see the bags under my eyes that are not errant eye liner. I see the lines in my faces, especially around my mouth, that weren't there just a year ago. I see the stubborn fat around my middle that frustrates me no end. I see that it takes me forever (okay, so I'm being figurative here, folks) to recover from the flu, and I see how easily I become – and stay – tired. The dancer in me screams, "No fair!" The adult patient in me says, "Deal with it," so I do.

I've used quite a bit of advanced terminology today, but haven't explained a great deal of it in the hopes that when you read these articles their meanings will become clear in context. If they don't, please leave me a comment and I will explore each one of them in future blogs. Who knows? Maybe I'll need to devote an entire blog to whichever term it is you'd like to know more about.

Don't let our premature aging get you down. We can work against it and, hopefully, slow it down just as we do with the progress of the decline in our kidney function.

I have been saving this bit of news for the last item in today's blog. The world is not going to suffer if it doesn't know about my photography, my teaching, writing, or acting careers. But, when it comes to CKD, my writing can add something for those 31 million people who have it...especially the 90% that haven't been diagnosed yet. What I did was completely change my web site so that it deals only with my Chronic Kidney Disease Awareness Advocacy (It's all caps because that's the way I think of it.) under the umbrella of *SlowItDownCKD*. I have to admit, I was surprised to see how active I've been in the last decade. It's different when you see your work listed all in one place. Take a look at gail-raegarwood.com and tell me what you think, would you?

6/26/17 *Gluten Free*

"...I started GF mid-April & my June lab work showed significant improvement. My next lab work is not until August, but I feel & look so much better, and because my BP dropped so much, my nephrologist took me off hydrochlorothorozide and reduced irbesartan from 300 to 75."

This is a small part of the message I received from a reader... and it intrigued me.

I take hydrochlorothiazide. I know I looked it up at the time it was prescribed, something about fluid. Hmmm, it wouldn't hurt to look it up again to refresh my (and your) memory. According to Medicinenet.com at http://www.medicinenet.com/hydrochlorothiazide/page2.htm, hydrochlorothiazide is prescribed for the following reasons:

"Hydrochlorothiazide is used to treat excessive fluid accumulation and swelling (edema) of the body caused by heart failure, cirrhosis, chronic kidney failure, corticosteroid medications, and nephrotic syndrome. It also is used alone or in conjunction with other blood pressure lowering medications to treat high blood pressure…. Hydrochlorothiazide can be used to treat calcium-containing kidney stones because it decreases the amount of calcium excreted by the kidneys in the urine and thus decreases the amount of calcium in urine to form stones…."

I didn't recognize irbesartan specifically, although the sartan part was familiar. According to the same source, but this time at http://www.medicinenet.com/irbesartan/article.htm,

"Irbesartan is used to treat high blood pressure (hypertension) and to help protect the kidneys from damage due to diabetes. Lowering high blood pressure helps prevent strokes, heart attacks, and kidney problems. Irbesartan belongs to a class of drugs called angiotensin receptor blockers (ARBs). It works by relaxing blood vessels so that blood can flow more easily."

Oh, of course! I'm taking losartan for the same reason. I'd had hypertension for over 20 years before I was diagnosed with Chronic Kidney Disease. Even if I hadn't, once I was diagnosed with CKD, a drug like this would have been prescribed. As a matter of fact, when I complained to my primary care doctor that I was taking too many pills (mostly supplements), she came up with one that combined hydrochlorothiazide and losartan.

But I digress. So, it's a good thing that this reader no longer needs her hydrochlorothiazide since she has no swelling and that her losartan has been reduced since her blood vessels are becoming more relaxed. Wait a minute. Why wouldn't every CKD patient want these results? Ah, but I've left something out of the equation.

She's gone GF or Gluten Free. Ready? Here is the definition of gluten from the Oxford Dictionary

"A mixture of two proteins present in cereal grains, especially wheat, which is responsible for the elastic texture of dough."

Oh, come on. There must be more to it than that. Let's try gluten free instead of gluten. Oh, my! NephCure at https://nephcure.org/livingwithkidneydisease/diet-and-nutrition/gluten-free-diet/ has an entire page devoted to going gluten free. But I am getting ahead of myself here.

Let's go back to gluten, this time sources. The American Diabetes Association offers these lists:

"What Foods Have Gluten?
Gluten is found in wheat, rye, barley and any foods made with these grains. Avoiding wheat can be especially hard because this means you should avoid all wheat-based flours and ingredients. These include but are not limited to:
White Flour
Whole Wheat Flour
Durum Wheat
Graham Flour
Triticale
Kamut
Semolina
Spelt
Wheat Germ
Wheat Bran
Common foods that are usually made with wheat include:
Pasta
Couscous
Bread
Flour Tortillas
Cookies
Cakes
Muffins
Pastries
Cereal
Crackers
Beer
Oats (see the section on oats below)
Gravy
Dressings
Sauces

This may seem like a long list, but there are still plenty of gluten-free foods out there! Choose from many fresh, healthy foods like fruits, vegetables, beans, dairy, nuts and gluten-free grains like quinoa or rice. There are also gluten-free versions of many of the foods above available in most grocery stores. You just have to look for them!

Gluten Surprises
You may not expect it, but the following foods can also contain gluten:
broth in soups and bouillon cubes
breadcrumbs and croutons
some candies
fried foods
imitation fish
some lunch meats and hot dogs
malt
matzo
modified food starch
seasoned chips and other seasoned snack foods
salad dressings
self-basting turkey
soy sauce
seasoned rice and pasta mixes

There are also many additives and ingredients in packaged foods that may contain gluten. Always check labels and ingredient lists for these. For a more comprehensive list of gluten-containing additives, contact your local celiac support group.

Other Tips to Remember
Don't forget that ingredients in food products change frequently, so always check the label before buying packaged foods. Remember that "wheat-free" does not automatically mean "gluten-free." While a product may not contain wheat, it can still contain rye or barley in some form. If you have any question about whether a food contains gluten, contact the manufacturer directly.

The Fuss About Oats
Pure oats are a gluten-free food, but most commercially processed oats have been contaminated during the growing, harvesting or processing stages. In the past, many experts recommended completely avoiding oats those on a gluten-free diet in addition to wheat, barley, and rye. Now, some oats are grown and processed separately, and can be labeled 'gluten-free.'"

I see an awful lot of the same foods to avoid on this list as I do on the renal diet. I wonder if that would make it easier to go gluten free if you decide to?

Phosphorous! Aha. We, as CKD patients, need to limit our phosphorous intake. Have you noticed that many of these foods are high phosphorous? Is it possible that the gluten free diet will help us with our renal diets? I'm not suggesting that you go gluten free and I'm not suggesting that you don't. I am saying the idea is, well, intriguing.

Before I forget: SlowItDownCKD has been chosen as one of Healthline's top kidney disease blogs for 2017. Second year in a row!!!!!

7/3/17 *Two Masters*

A friend of mine, the one I mentioned when I wrote about renal sally ports, recently has had a relapse. Yep, he neglected to take his medications at the proper times. That can cause havoc for mental illness, especially bipolar disorder. It got me to thinking. What if my friend had Chronic Kidney Disease AND bipolar disease? How could he handle both diagnoses at the same time?

Let's start at the beginning. There are certain drugs I take in the hopes of delaying dialysis as long as possible. One of those is the ACE Inhibitor I'd been taking for hypertension for about two decades before I was even diagnosed with CKD. Here's the definition from **What Is It and How Did I Get It? Early Stage Chronic Kidney Disease**:

"ACE Inhibitor: A blood pressure medication that lowers protein in the urine if you have CKD."

It works by both relaxing the blood vessels and reducing the blood volume. This, in turn, lowers your blood pressure which, in turn, lowers your heart's oxygen needs. And the problem for my friend would be? Well, maybe just remembering to take the medication each day.

However, according to Medicine Net, the most common side effects are:
• Cough
• Elevated blood potassium levels
• Low blood pressure
• Dizziness
• Headache
• Drowsiness
• Weakness
• Abnormal taste (metallic or salty taste)

- Rash
- Chest pain
- Increased uric acid levels
- Sun sensitivity
- Increased BUN and creatinine levels

Did you notice increased uric acid levels, and increased BUN and creatinine levels? This could be a dicey medication for CKD patients if they did not heed their doctor's advice once (s)he has evaluated the patient's labs. That's the problem here: not having the ability to be a compliant patient during a bipolar episode.
I was also prescribed a drug for cholesterol, a statin. This drug inhibits (the word of the day) an enzyme in the liver that produces lipids. As reported in *The Book of Blogs: Moderate Stage Chronic Kidney Disease, Part 1*:

According to Dr. Dr. Robert Provenzano, chief of nephrology at St. John Hospital and Medical Center in Detroit, "...LDL, bad cholesterol, directly impacts acceleration of Chronic Kidney Disease."

One of the possible side effects is of this drug is Type 2 Diabetes. All I can say about that is thank goodness these side effects are not the norm.

Here's the problem: statins have to be taken at night. That's when the body produces cholesterol. Again, can my friend be compliant during an episode? What about the drugs he already takes? Are they going to somehow interfere with these common drugs for CKD?

Lithium is the usual drug for him. This is from *The Book of Blogs: Moderate Stage Chronic Kidney Disease, Part 2*:

"There were two Plenary Sessions I attended at the Southwest Nephrology Conference I attended last weekend. It was at the second one, 'Psychiatric issues in kidney patients' that I suddenly sprang to attention. What was this man saying? Something about lithium doubling the risk for Chronic Kidney Disease? And I was off... how many psychiatric patients knew that fact? How many of their caretakers knew that just in case the patient was not responsible at the time of treatment? What about children? Did their parents know? Was a screening for CKD performed BEFORE lithium was prescribed?"

Kidney.org at https://www.kidney.org/atoz/content/lithium has me downright frightened for my friend:

"What is lithium?
Lithium is a common medicine used to help calm mood for treating people with mental disorders. Since such disorders need life-long treatment, long-term use of lithium may be harmful to organs, such as the kidneys.

How does lithium cause kidney damage?
Lithium may cause problems with kidney health. Kidney damage due to lithium may include acute (sudden) or chronic (long-term) kidney disease and kidney cysts. The amount of kidney damage depends on how long you have been taking lithium. It is possible to reverse kidney damage caused by lithium early in treatment, but the damage may become permanent over time.

What is nephrogenic diabetes insipidus?
The most common problem from taking lithium is a form of diabetes due to kidney damage called nephrogenic diabetes insipidus. This type of diabetes is different than diabetes mellitus caused by high blood sugar. In nephrogenic diabetes insipidus, the kidneys cannot respond to anti-diuretic hormone (ADH), a chemical messenger that controls fluid balance. This results in greater than normal urine out-put and excessive thirst. It can be hard to treat nephrogenic diabetes insipidus."

I keep reminding myself that the word "may" appears over and over again. Yet, since my friend either wasn't taking his medication at all or not taking it as prescribed, it wasn't working...and he is still at risk for CKD.

I found this tidbit on Drugs.com at https://www.drugs.com/interactions-check.php?drug_list=1477-0,1489-0, ACE Inhibitors:
"...may increase the blood levels and effects of lithium. You may need a dose adjustment or more frequent monitoring by your doctor to safely use both medications."

Wait. So you need an ACE Inhibitor if you have CKD, but it can interfere with the lithium you take if you're bi-polar. And statins? While I couldn't find any interactions, I did find the caution that there may be some and to check with your doctor. I am aware he takes an anti-depressant, but in researching, have discovered there are many that are safe to take with CKD.

My friend usually goes to his medical appointments, but he neglects to mention certain symptoms and sometimes has trouble telling reality from non-reality. Does he know whether his doctor has warned him about the higher risk of CKD or not? Does he know that he may develop a form of diabetes from long term use of lithium? Does he know that if even one of his parents has CKD, his risk is doubled yet again?

Tomorrow is July 4th, the day the United States celebrates its independence from the tyranny of England. Where is my friend's independence from the tyranny of his mental illness? The English and the United States have learned to peacefully share our existences (right, English readers?). Here's hoping my friend can learn to peacefully share his existence with bipolar disorder... and CKD should he develop it. Heaven forbid.

7/10/17 *Updated*

You may have seen the pictures of the updates we've been making to our home on Facebook or Instagram. Now, it seemed to me
that if I could update my home, I could update **SlowItDownCKD**'s
social media. So I did. The website at gail-raegarwood.com is totally **SlowItDownCKD** now, as are the Instagram, LinkedIn, Twitter,
and Pinterest accounts. Of course, the blog was next. I liked my
updates, but realized some of the new organizations on the blogroll (the list to the right of the blog) may be unknown to you.
No problem. I'll just introduce them to you. Allow me to make the
introductions…

We'll go alphabetically down the roll here. The **American Association of Kidney Patients**, The **American Kidney Fund**, and The
American Society of Nephrology are not new. Just in case you
need a reminder of what each is, I've linked their titles to the organization. Just click on one of them to go to their websites, as
you usually do for any title on the blogroll.

This brings us to **The International Federation of Kidney Foundations**. This is directly from the young (established 1999) organization's website:

"**The International Federation of Kidney Foundations** leads the
way in the prevention and treatment of kidney disease, through
its Membership on all continents around the world. The Federation was formed to foster international collaboration and the exchange of ideas that will improve the health, well-being and quality of life of individuals with kidney disease. We hope to achieve
this by advocating for improved health care delivery as well as
adopting and disseminating standards of best practice of treatment and care. We facilitate education programs for member or-
ganisations, promote research, communicate with other organisa-

tions and exchange ideas, particularly those concerning fund raising....

The IFKF helps facilitate the establishment of more kidney foundations and to help existing foundations become more dynamic and effective. Worldwide, most individuals with chronic kidney disease or hypertension are not diagnosed until long after the illness has developed. Moreover, when they are diagnosed they are too often treated sub-optimally or not at all. In many parts of the world, once end stage kidney failure occurs, patients do not have access to dialysis or kidney transplantation.

IFKF members join together with ISN members and kidney patient associations, to celebrate World Kidney Day annually in March, to influence general physicians, primary healthcare providers, health officials and policymakers and to educate high risk patients and individuals."

I've been interested in the global effects of Chronic Kidney Disease since I started preparing for Landmark's 2017 Conference for Global Transformation at which I presented this past May. Writing two articles for their journal opened my eyes- yet again – to the fact that this is not just a local problem, but a worldwide problem. That's why I included Kidney Diseases Death Rate By Country, On a World Map in the blogroll. I mapped out the statistics I found here on a trifold map to exhibit at the conference. Seeing the numbers spread all over the world was startling, to say the least.
Here is their 2015 global CKD information:

"In 2015, the Asian nations of India and China fared the worst when it came to the number of deaths due to this degenerative health condition per thousand people. According to the World Health Organization (WHO) data *(I'm interrupting. Would you like a link to WHO on the blogroll?)*, India had the highest number of kidney diseases deaths. The data put the figure at an astounding

257.9 per 1,000 people. China had the second highest number of deaths due to kidney diseases. Here, the number stood at 187.4 per 1,000 people. Though not as bad as the two Asian nations, the United States was also grappling with the problem of kidney diseases deaths in 2015. The nation had 59.8 deaths (per 1,000 people) due to kidney diseases, while Indonesia, which occupied the fourth place, had an estimated 43 deaths (per 1,000 people) due to kidney diseases. Nations such as Egypt, Germany, Mexico, Philippines, Brazil, Thailand and Japan reported deaths between 20 and 40 (per 1,000 people) due to kidney-related diseases. But, on the positive side, there were many nations in the world where a negligible number of people died due to kidney diseases. It is a noteworthy fact that countries such as Maldives, Vanuatu, Iceland, Grenada, Comoros, Belize, and many others, reported a zero figure in 2015."

But then I wanted to cover more localized information about CKD, so I included The National Chronic Kidney Disease, Fact Sheet, 2017. This is basically facts with pictograms that make the information about the United States' CKD information more visual and easier to grasp. The information is more distressing each year the site is updated.

Fast Stats
• 30 million people or 15% of US adults are estimated to have CKD.*
• 48% of those with severely reduced kidney function but not on dialysis are not aware of having CKD.
• Most (96%) people with kidney damage or mildly reduced kidney function are not aware of having CKD.

After several sites that are not new, the last new site, other than direct links to **SlowItDownCKD**'s kidney books, is The Kidney & Urology Foundation of America. Why did I include that? Take a look at their website. You'll find this there:

"**The Kidney & Urology Foundation** focuses on care and support of the patient, the concerns of those at risk, education for the community and medical professionals, methods of prevention, and improved treatment options.

What Sets Us Apart?
The Kidney & Urology Foundation of America is comprised of a dedicated Executive Board, medical advisors, educated staff and volunteers who provide individualized support to patients and their families. Adult nephrologists and transplant physicians comprise our Medical Advisory Board, Board – certified urologists serve on the Urology Board, and pediatric nephrologists and urologists represent the Council on Pediatric Nephrology and Urology. We are a phone call or e-mail click away from getting you the help you need to cope with a new diagnosis, a resource for valuable information on kidney or urologic diseases, a window into current research treatment options or a link to a physician should you need one."

Are there any organizations I've left out that you feel should be included? Just add a comment and I'll be glad to take a look at them. I am convinced that the only way we're going to get any kind of handle on Chronic Kidney Disease as patients is by keeping each other updated.

7/17/17 *Singapore Knows CKD*

I have an online friend, Leong Seng Chen, who lives in Singapore and is highly active in the Chronic Kidney Disease Awareness community there. Last week, I asked if any readers would like to see certain organizations that weren't already there added to the blogroll – the list of CKD organizations to the right of the blog itself. He mentioned two but one was a Facebook page and the other was for dialysis. I usually write a blog about current Facebook pages once a year and don't usually write about dialysis. His request, which I couldn't honor, got me to thinking about what is going on for CKD patients in Singapore. So, I started poking around.

The Clinical Journal of the American Society of Nephrology (of all places!) looked into this in 2008, a decade ago, and published the following at http://cjasn.asnjournals.org/content/3/2/610.full.

The NKF Singapore Prevention Program presents a unique approach that incorporates a comprehensive multilevel strategy to address chronic kidney disease …. What makes the NKF Singapore program different is that it incorporated a public health approach to preventing ESRD by using primary, secondary, and tertiary prevention initiatives that can intervene at several stages in the progression of kidney disease. These include 1) surveillance of the general population for urinary abnormalities, 2) screening of the general population for clinical conditions that increase the risk of chronic kidney disease, such as diabetes mellitus and hypertension, 3) the institution of a disease management program to facilitate the management of patients with diabetes and hypertension, which are among the leading causes of ESRD in the country, and to a limited extent, 4) tracking of the individuals who participate in the screening program. Thus, both population-based and high-risk prevention strategies were incorporated into the Singapore Prevention Program.

If you think about it for a moment, this is an astoundingly comprehensive approach to awareness, prevention, and treatment. I was intrigued and looked further. I had naively assumed the National Kidney Foundation was an American organization. Here, in the United States, it is. There, in Singapore, it's a Singaporean organization.

In Singapore, CKD awareness is not just an adult undertaking. There is a bus provided by the NKF that goes to schools, among other places, to educate young children about how to prevent and recognize the disease, as well as what the kidneys do. Somehow, I found that charming and necessary simultaneously. Why don't we do that in the United States, I wonder. Take a look at https://www.nkfs.org/kidney-health-education-bus/ to see for yourself what I'm talking about here.

The National Registry of Disease Office was founded by the Ministry of Health in 2001. While the most current statistics I could find, they only record Chronic Kidney Failure, or End Stage Chronic Renal Disease (ESRD). According to their website at https://www.nrdo.gov.sg/about-us,

"We are responsible for:
• collecting the data and maintaining the registry on reportable health conditions and diseases that have been diagnosed and treated in Singapore
• publishing reports on these health conditions and diseases
• providing information to support national public health policies, healthcare services and programmes,"

Meanwhile, the statistics from Global Disease Burden at Health Grove are only four years old and give us a better understanding of what's happening in Singapore as far as CKD. As they phrase it:

"These risk factors contributed to, and were thought to be responsible for, an estimated 100% of the total deaths caused by chronic kidney disease in Singapore during 2013."

I hadn't been aware of just how involved with CKD Singapore is until Leong started telling me. Now, I'm astounded to learn that this country is number four in deaths from our disease.

Just as in the United States, Singapore posts lists of nephrologists, herbal aids, hospital studies, and even medical tourism sites.

While I may or may not approve of such listings, they have opened my eyes to the fact that Singapore plays with the big boys when it comes to CKD. Come to think of it, they may even be more developed when it comes to educating the public. Remember those education buses?

Many thanks to Leong Seng Chen, my CKD friend on Facebook this past year and- hopefully – many more years to come.

Before I forget:
Did you know that the Kindle versions of each of the *SlowItDownCKD* books is now $2.99 in order make them more accessible to more people. I'm working on lowering the price for the print books on Amazon.com, too, but that seems to be more complicated...or maybe I just don't understand the process yet.

By the way, have you heard about this from AAKP? (You can read more about it on their website.)

AAKP has been in the news and across social media lately as public interest continues to build in KidneyWorks – a groundbreaking national initiative we developed in full collaboration with our partners at the Medical Education Institute (MEI). The multiphase initiative aims to identify and address barriers to continued employment for individuals with chronic kidney disease (CKD). Phase I of KidneyWorks involved a consensus roundtable of national experts on kidney disease and workforce experts who convened in Washington, D.C. and the development and public release of a White Paper detailing strategies to help working-age people with non-dialysis chronic kidney disease (CKD) improve their lives, slow CKD progression, and keep their jobs. Phases II and III will involve the development, production and dissemination of strategies and online and mobile tools that help workers, caregivers and employers help achieve the goals of KidneyWorks.

7/24/17 *Shocked*

When I checked my phone messages this morning, I saw one from
the wife of someone I have known and loved my whole life. That
shook me. The message was from his wife, not him. I couldn't
bring myself to listen to it until after I'd had a cup of coffee and
fed Shiloh, our dog.

It was bad news. He was in the hospital on life support. I was
shocked. Immediately, I felt nausea and a band started to tighten
around my head. I noticed my voice was rough as I tried to process what his wife was telling me.

She did an exemplary job of explaining what had happened step
by step and including what will happen at the hospital now. After
reassuring myself that she had friends around her to support her
while she's emergency central, so to speak, we hung up...and I
tried to go through my usual early morning routines.

I knew it wasn't working when I took the wash out of washing machine, put it back in the washing machine, and started the empty
dryer. I knew it wasn't working when I fed the dog I'd just fed.
So I retreated to the library to start the daily 'kidney work': check-
ing email, texts, and LinkedIn for messages from readers; posting
on Instagram and Facebook; and perusing Twitter for articles that
might interest you. I was having trouble concentrating. Maybe
thinking about what I'd write in today's blog would be more productive.

It was obvious, wasn't it? I'd write about what shock does to your
body and to your kidneys.

In befuddedly casting around on the internet for information, I
found this at http://www.harleytherapy.co.uk/counselling/7-
warning-signs-acute-stress-reaction-emotional-shock.htm.

By Harley Therapy January 23, 2014 Anxiety & stress, Counselling

…. While it's true you aren't in "medical shock" – an acute circulatory condition where blood pressure falls so severely that multiple organ failure can occur – you are still in a medically recognised kind of shock.

Psychological shock, a form of psychological trauma, is the body's very real stress response to experiencing or witnessing an overwhelming and/or frightening event….

You might feel as if your brain has turned to mush, or you have 'brain fog'….

Life might even feel unreal, as if you are disconnected, floating slightly outside of your body and watching yourself carry on doing things. This is called dissociation….

When your brain decides that there is 'danger' around, it triggers the primal 'fight, flight, or flight' response. Back when we were 'cave people' these responses where helpful, but nowadays the overload of adrenaline they involve just leave you with a racing heartbeat, muscle tension, headaches, stomach upset, and random aches and pains….

Sleep is often affected by emotional shock. Insomnia is common. Even if you are sleeping more than ever, you are unlikely to get quality sleep but might suffer disturbed sleep, full of stress dreams. It's common to develop 'night panic attacks' where you wake up suddenly with a racing heart and severe anxiety….

I could identify with this. It seemed I had to correct the spelling of every other word today. My husband was trying to pin down dates for a California trip and I was responding with dates for a New York trip. The doorbell rang, so I answered the phone. You get the idea. I've already mentioned the particular headache and the nausea. But what about my kidneys? What was happening to them?

The Medical Dictionary at http://medical-dictionary.thefreedictionary.com/shock+organs, defines shock as

"a sudden disturbance of mental equilibrium."

That is a pretty accurate description of what happened when I returned that phone call this morning.

The same site goes on to explain that shock
"is associated with a dangerously low blood pressure."

And blood pressure, of course is:

pressure that is exerted by the blood upon the walls of the blood vessels and especially arteries and that varies with the muscular efficiency of the heart, the blood volume and viscosity, the age and health of the individual, and the state of the vascular wall

Thank you to the Merriam-Webster Dictionary at https://www.merriam- web-ster.com/dictionary/blood%20pressure for that definition.

Notice the word "arteries." Arteries also run into the kidneys. The following is from *What Is It and How Did I Get It? Early Stage Chronic Kidney Disease.*

Your kidneys have about a million nephrons, which are those tiny structures that produce urine as part of the body's waste removal process. Each of them has a glomerulus or network of capillaries. This is where the blood from the renal artery is filtered.
In other words, when you're in shock – even if it's emotional shock – the pressure of your blood can be dangerously low. But

121

low blood pressure may also lead to Acute Kidney Injury (AKI). Uh-oh, I remember writing about that in *The Book of Blogs: Moderate Stage Chronic Kidney Disease, Part 2.*

....Chronic Kidney Disease is a risk factor for acute kidney injury, acute kidney injury is a risk factor for the development of Chronic Kidney Disease, and both acute kidney injury and Chronic Kidney Disease are risk factors for cardiovascular disease.... Not surprisingly, the risk factors for AKI {Once again, that's acute kidney injury.} are the same as those for CKD... except for one peculiar circumstance. Having CKD itself can raise the risk of AKI 10 times. Whoa! If you're Black, of an advanced age {Hey!}, or have diabetes, you already know you're at risk for CKD, or are the one out of nine in our country that has it. Once you've developed CKD, you've just raised the risk for AKI 10 times.

Let me make sure you (and I) understand that this is the worst case scenario. A few thoughts about how cardiovascular disease and the kidneys interact before I get on the phone to check on my beloved friend again. This is from a study that was included in *The Book of Blogs: Moderate Stage Chronic Kidney Disease, Part 1.*

"The brain and kidney are both organs that are affected by the cardiovascular systems," said the study's lead author, Adam Davey, associate professor of public health in Temple's College of Health Professions and Social Work. "They are both affected by things like blood pressure and hypertension, so it is natural to expect that changes in one organ are going to be linked with changes in another."

8/7/17 *Long Term, Short, and your Heart*

It seems Acute Kidney Disease (AKI) is a new topic for so many of us. By us I mean Chronic Kidney Disease (CKD) patients. I know at stage 3, my nephrologist never brought this up to me.

Ah, but I remembered this from *The Book of Blogs: Moderate Stage Chronic Kidney Disease, Part 2*:

"On the very first page of *What Is It and How Did I Get It? Early Stage Chronic Kidney Disease*, I wrote

'...chronic is not acute. It means long term, whereas acute usually means quick onset and short duration.'"

All those years of teaching English in high school and college paid off for me right there in that sentence.

I'd always thought that AKI and CKD were separate issues and I'll bet you did, too. But Dr. L.S. Chawla and his co-writers based the following conclusion on the labor of epidemiologists and others. (Note: Dr. Chawla et al wrote a review article in the *New England Journal of Medicine* in 2014.)

"Chronic Kidney Disease is a risk factor for acute kidney injury, acute kidney injury is a risk factor for the development of Chronic Kidney Disease, and both acute kidney injury and Chronic Kidney Disease are risk factors for cardiovascular disease...."

Not surprisingly, the risk factors for AKI {Once again, that's acute kidney injury.} are the same as those for CKD... except for one peculiar circumstance. Having CKD itself can raise the risk of AKI 10 times. Whoa! If you're Black, of an advanced age {Hey!}, or have diabetes, you already know you're at risk for CKD, or are the one out of nine in our country that has it. Once you've developed CKD, you've just raised the risk for AKI 10 times. I'm getting a little nervous here....

It makes sense, as researchers and doctors are beginning to see, that these are all connected. I'm not a doctor or a researcher, but I can understand that if you've had some kind of insult to your kidney, it would be more apt to develop CKD.

And the CVD risk? Let's think of it this way. You've had AKI. That period of weakness in the kidneys opens them up to CKD. We already know there's a connection between CKD and CVD. Throw that AKI into the mix, and you have more of a chance to develop CVD whether or not you've had a problem in this area before. Let's not go off the deep end here. If you've had AKI, you just need to be monitored to see if CKD develops and avoid nephrotoxic {Kidney poisoning} medications such as NSAIDS... contrast dyes, and radioactive substances. This is just so circular! As with CKD, your hypertension and diabetes {If you have them.} need to be monitored, too. Then there's the renal diet, especially low sodium foods. The kicker here is that no one knows if this is helpful in avoiding CKD after an AKI... it's a 'just in case' kind of thing to help ward off any CKD and possible CVD from the CKD. Has your primary care doctor recommended a daily low dose aspirin with your nephrologist's approval? This is to protect your heart against CVD since you already have CKD which raises the risk of CVD. Now here's where it gets confusing, the FDA has recently revoked its endorsement of such a regiment.

Let's see what more we can find out about this dastardly triumvirate. The National Kidney Foundation at https://www.kidney.org/atoz/content/AcuteKidneyInjury offers this information about AKI.

"Acute kidney injury (AKI) is a sudden episode of kidney failure or kidney damage that happens within a few hours or a few days. AKI causes a build-up of waste products in your blood and makes it hard for your kidneys to keep the right balance of fluid in your body. AKI can also affect other organs such as the brain, heart, and lungs. Acute kidney injury is common in patients who are in the hospital, in intensive care units, and especially in older adults."

You did catch that it can affect the heart, right? Well, what about the heart and its diseases? This is from the Mayo Clinic at http://www.mayoclinic.org/diseases-conditions/heart-disease/basics/definition/con-20034056.

"The term 'heart disease' is often used interchangeably with the term 'cardiovascular disease.'

Cardiovascular disease generally refers to conditions that involve narrowed or blocked blood vessels that can lead to a heart attack, chest pain (angina) or stroke. Other heart conditions, such as those that affect your heart's muscle, valves or rhythm, also are considered forms of heart disease.

Many forms of heart disease can be prevented or treated with healthy lifestyle choices."

Maybe a reminder of what CKD is will help, too. WebMD at http://www.webmd.com/a-to-z-guides/tc/chronic-kidney-disease-topic-overview#1 offers this simple, comprehensive explanation.

"Having chronic kidney disease means that for some time your kidneys have not been working the way they should. Your kidneys have the important job of filtering your blood. They remove waste products and extra fluid and flush them from your body as urine. When your kidneys don't work right, wastes build up in your blood and make you sick.

Chronic kidney disease may seem to have come on suddenly. But it has been happening bit by bit for many years as a result of damage to your kidneys.

Each of your kidneys has about a million tiny filters, called nephrons. If nephrons are damaged, they stop working. For a while, healthy nephrons can take on the extra work. But if the damage continues, more and more nephrons shut down. After a certain point, the nephrons that are left cannot filter your blood well enough to keep you healthy."

My head is spinning. One could – or could not – lead to another which, in turn, could – or could not – lead to the third. There's no strict order and there's no way of knowing until you actually have it. My layperson's suggestion? Take good care of your kidneys

8/14/17 *Good Grief!*

No, Charlie Brown, grief is not good. Grief is not good at all. My big brother, Alan Peckolick, died 10 days ago. You can read about him in lots of publications and I'll even provide the links.* But you can't read about him as my big brother in any of these.

But I found myself grieving. It was not unexpected. I hurt all over, nothing specific, just a general aching… or was it my heart I felt aching? Wait a minute, what was happening to my kidneys throughout this process of grief?

The day he was taken off life support, I was at my lab having the usual quarterly blood draw. Alan and Jessica Weber, his wife, were in Connecticut where they have a country house and where the catastrophic fall that landed him on life support occurred; I was in Arizona. There was nothing I could do from afar and I knew I could trust Jessica to keep me informed. I thought keeping myself to my usual schedule would help me cope.

Except for the values in the next sentence, all my tests came back as low as they could while still being in the normal range. That had never happened before: while my GFR stayed stable, my BUN was at 30 ('normal' range is 8-25), n/Creatinine Ratio 29.1 ('normal' range is 10-28) and my glucose was 113 ('normal' range is 65-99). I was underwhelmed. I figured it was my brother's situation making my body goes haywire. I still am.

PyschCentral at https://psychcentral.com/lib/your-health-and-grief/ offers the following explanation of how grief affects our bodies:

"…. At the death the brain 'translates' the stress of grief into a chemical reaction in the body. The pituitary gland located at the base of the brain is stimulated to produce a hormone called adrenocorticotrophin hormone (ACTH). This reaction is a 'protective' one and in essence makes the body ready to do battle. The ACTH (from the pituitary gland) then travels to the adrenal gland, a gland at the top of the kidneys, which causes a chemical reaction which ultimately produces cortisone. As the cortisone level increases it causes the production of ACTH to level off.

What happens in the case of grief where the stress continues for many months? The cycle does not operate as it should. Because the stress is continuing, the production of ACTH is continuing thus causing the adrenal gland to produce more and more cortisone. The result is an abnormally high level of cortisone circulating in the blood sometimes exceeding ten to twenty times the normal levels.

A high level of cortisone is one of the things that causes our immune system (the system that normally fights off disease carrying bacteria fungi and viruses) to falter. The high level of cortisone affects yet another gland the thalamus which manufactures the white cells of our blood. With the thalamus not functioning properly, it cannot produce white cells that are effective. Those white cells normally locate and phagocytize (eat up) the invading germs, viral particles or even pre-cancerous cells. Thus with the white cells unable to function properly the individual is 100% more susceptible to the most common germs."

Well, what is cortisol? As I mentioned in *SlowItDownCKD 2016*,

"Cortisol is a hormone that controls metabolism and helps the body react to stress, according to EndocrineWeb. It affects the immune system and lowers inflammatory responses in the body."

So our already compromised immune system is compromised even more compromised. Are we now at the mercy of our grief? Nothing that dramatic, folks.

We can up our vitamin D – with our nephrologist's approval first, of course. As mentioned in the glossary of *What Is It and How Did I Get It? Early Stage Chronic Kidney Disease*,

"Vitamin D: Regulates calcium and phosphorous blood levels as well as promoting bone formation, among other tasks – affects the immune system."

We can up our NREM (non-rapid eye movement) sleep. I turned to *The Book of Blogs: Moderate Stage Chronic Kidney Disease, Part 2* for this information:

"WebMD tells us

During the deep stages of NREM sleep, the body repairs and re-generates tissues, builds bone and muscle, and appears to strengthen the immune system."

My favorite deterrent to a further compromised immune system? Hugs. MedicalNewsToday explains:

"Oxytocin has an anti-anxiety (anxiolytic) effect …."
Less anxiety, less stress. That's something that could be useful during times of grief. I didn't have to clear this with my nephrologist, hugging is a way of life with my family and friends, and it somehow, magically, lessens the pain for a little while.

8/21/17 *I'll Sleep When I'm Dead*

How many times have you said this (before your diagnose) to those who told you to slow down, take it easier, don't rush so, take some time for yourself, etc.? As a younger person, I was a high school teacher, an actor, a writer, and – most importantly – a mother, actually a single mother once my daughters were double digit aged.

Guess what. You may sleep when you're dead, but you need to sleep now before you hasten the time to your death. What's that? You get enough sleep? I thought I did, too, but I wasn't getting the kind of sleep I needed.

Why do we need sleep anyway? I turned to **The Book of Blogs: Moderate Stage Chronic Kidney Disease, Part 1** for some answers. The first reason I stumbled across was in an article from *The Journal of The American Society of Nephrologists*:

"Hermida tells WebMD that some of the body's blood pressure control systems are most active while we sleep. So medicines designed to control those systems work better when taken close to the time when the systems are activated most fully."

Ramon C. Hermida, PhD is the director of the bioengineering and chronobiology labs at the University of Vigo in Spain.

Hmmm, I take medication for hypertension... and I take it at night. I see that I need to sleep for it to work most effectively. I've known this for years and written about it. The point is you may need to know about it.

Then I started wondering if I were correct in the amount of sleep I thought I needed. **The Book of Blogs: Moderate Stage Chronic Kidney Disease, Part 2** was helpful here:

"How much sleep is enough sleep anyway? According to Dr. Timothy Morgenthaler of The Mayo Clinic site, seven to eight hours is what an adult needs, but then he lists mitigating circumstances under which you might need more:

• Pregnancy. Changes in a woman's body during early pregnancy can increase the need for sleep.
• Aging. Older adults need about the same amount of sleep as younger adults. As you get older, however, your sleeping patterns might change. Older adults tend to sleep more lightly and for shorter time spans than do younger adults. This might create a need for spending more time in bed to get enough sleep, or a tendency toward daytime napping.
• Previous sleep deprivation. If you're sleep deprived, the amount of sleep you need increases.
• Sleep quality. If your sleep is frequently interrupted or cut short, you're not getting quality sleep. The quality of your sleep is just as important as the quantity."

While I'm not pregnant (and will become a medical miracle if I become pregnant), all the other circumstances do apply to me. During Shiva - the week long period of mourning observed by first degree relatives in the Jewish religion -after my brother's death, there was very, very little sleeping going on. Hence, sleep deprivation. I'm aging and my sleep quality is not great right now. Those are my circumstances, but they could be yours. Are you getting enough sleep?

Sometimes, simply having Chronic Kidney Disease can be the source of sleep problems. This is something I've written about several times. Here's an excerpt from *SlowItDownCKD 2015* about just that:

'"We've known for a long time that sleep disorders are more common in kidney disease patients than in the general population,' Charles Atwood, MD, associate director of the University of Pittsburgh Medical Center's Sleep Medicine Center in Pennsylvania, who wasn't involved in the study, told Medscape Medical News. 'A lot of studies in the past focused on the dialysis population. It seems like this group focused on people with milder degrees of kidney disease and basically found that they also have sleep disorders and I'm not surprised by that,' he added."

By digging deep, far and wide, I finally figured out that toxic waste buildup in our systems (from the imperfect blood filtering by our kidneys) could be the cause of my segmented sleep. I took a comment from one study, a sentence from another, and unilaterally decided this was the reason. I am not a doctor – as I keep saying – and I don't have the facts I'd like to behind this conclusion...."

Oh, right: you need a definition of segmented sleep. Wikipedia provides one:

"Segmented sleep, also known as divided sleep, bimodal sleep pattern, bifurcated sleep, or interrupted sleep, is a polyphasic or biphasic sleep pattern where two or more periods of sleep are punctuated by periods of wakefulness."

The National Institutes of Health at https://www.nhlbi.nih.gov/health/health-topics/topics/sdd/why sums up our need for sleep beautifully:

"Sleep plays an important role in your physical health. For example, sleep is involved in healing and repair of your heart and blood vessels. Ongoing sleep deficiency is linked to an increased risk of heart disease, kidney disease, high blood pressure, diabetes, and stroke.

Sleep deficiency also increases the risk of obesity. For example, one study of teenagers showed that with each hour of sleep lost, the odds of becoming obese went up. Sleep deficiency increases the risk of obesity in other age groups as well.

Sleep helps maintain a healthy balance of the hormones that make you feel hungry (ghrelin) or full (leptin). When you don't get enough sleep, your level of ghrelin goes up and your level of leptin goes down. This makes you feel hungrier than when you're well-rested.

Sleep also affects how your body reacts to insulin, the hormone that controls your blood glucose (sugar) level. Sleep deficiency results in a higher than normal blood sugar level, which may increase your risk for diabetes.

Sleep also supports healthy growth and development. Deep sleep triggers the body to release the hormone that promotes normal growth in children and teens. This hormone also boosts muscle mass and helps repair cells and tissues in children, teens, and adults. Sleep also plays a role in puberty and fertility.

Your immune system relies on sleep to stay healthy. This system defends your body against foreign or harmful substances. Ongoing sleep deficiency can change the way in which your immune system responds. For example, if you're sleep deficient, you may have trouble fighting common infections."

I think I need to go to sleep now.

8/28/17 *It's the Heat AND the Humidity*

Hawaii is so beautiful... and Maui so healing. There was just one thing, though. I somehow managed to forget how humid it is. As you may or may not remember, after we'd come back from the Caribbean and from San Antonio last year, I vowed never to go to a humid climate during the summer again. Well, Maui *was* Bear's 71st birthday present so maybe that's why I so conveniently forgot my vow.

Here's why I shouldn't have. This is updated from *SlowItDownCKD 2016*.

"ResearchGate at https://www.researchgate.net/publication/263084331_Climate change and Chronic Kidney Disease published a study from the *Asian Journal of Pharmaceutical and Clinical Research* from February of 2014 (That's over three years ago, friends.) which included the following in the conclusion:

'Our data suggest that burden of renal diseases may increase as period of hot weather becomes more frequent. This is further aggravated if age advanced and people with chronic diseases like diabetes and hypertension.'"

That makes sense, but how will this happen exactly? I included this June, 2010, article in *The Book of Blogs: Moderate Chronic Kidney Disease, Part 1*. Apparently, heat (and humidity) has been an acknowledged threat to our kidneys for longer than we'd thought.

"....Dr. HL Trivedi of the Institute of Kidney Diseases and Research Centre (IKDRC) said, '.... Rapid water loss causes the kidney's functioning to slow down, resulting in temporary or permanent kidney failure.' Extreme heat causes rapid water loss, resulting in acute electrolyte imbalance. The kidney, unable to cope with the water loss, fails to flush out the requisite amount of Creatinine and other toxins from the body. Coupled with a lack of consistent water intake, this brings about permanent or temporary kidney failure, explain experts.'"

The article can be viewed directly at http://www.dnaindia.com/health/report_heat-induced-kidney-ailments-see-40pct-rise_1390589 and is from Daily News & Analysis.

By the time this book's twin, *The Book of Blogs: Moderate Chronic Kidney Disease, Part 2*, was ready for publication, the (then) spokesman for The *National Kidney Foundation* – Dr. Leslie Spry – had this to say about heat and humidity:

"Heat illness occurs when body temperature exceeds a person's ability to dissipate that heat and is commonly diagnosed when the body temperature approaches 104 degrees Fahrenheit and when humidity is greater than 70 percent. Once the humidity is that high, sweating becomes less effective at dispersing body heat, and the core body temperature begins to rise."

The entire article is at http://www.huffingtonpost.com/leslie-spry-md-facp/heat-illness_b_1727995.html.

Oh, so humidity affects sweating and body heat rises. Humidity greater than 70%. That covers almost the entire time we were in the Caribbean and Texas (and now Hawaii). Well, what's the connection between heat illness and CKD then?

The CDC offers the following advice to avoid heat illness: "People with a chronic medical condition are less likely to sense and respond to changes in temperature. Also, they may be taking

medications that can worsen the impact of extreme heat. People in this category need the following information.
• Drink more water than usual and don't wait until you're thirsty to drink.
• Check on a friend or neighbor, and have someone do the same for you.
• Check the local news for health and safety updates regularly.
• Don't use the stove or oven to cook——it will make you and your house hotter.
• Wear loose, lightweight, light-colored clothing.
• Take cool showers or baths to cool down...."

Uh-oh, we're already in trouble. Look at the first suggestion: our fluid intake is restricted to 64 oz. (Mine is, check with your nephrologist for yours.) I know I carefully space out my fluids – which include anything that can melt to a liquid – to cover my entire day. I can't drink more water than usual and, sometimes – on those rare occasions when I've been careless – have to wait until I'm thirsty to drink.

Diabetes is the foremost cause of CKD. I was curious how heat affected blood sugar so I popped over to Information about Diabetes at
http://www.informationaboutdiabetes.com/lifestyle/lifestyle/how-heat-and-humidity-may-affect-blood-sugar and found this:

"1. If our body is low on fluids, the kidneys receive less blood flow and work less effectively. This might cause blood glucose concentrations to rise.
2. If someone's blood sugar is already running high in the heat, not only will they lose water through sweat but they might urinate more frequently too, depleting their body's fluids even more."
There's more at the website if this interests you.

According to the U.S. Department of Veterans' Affairs at https://www.visn9.va.gov/VISN9/news/vhw/summer07/humidity.asp,

"Hot weather can lead to dehydration, heat exhaustion and heat stroke, but the dangers increase when you add humidity to the mix. When the temperature rises above 70F and the humidity registers more than 70 percent, you need to be on the alert.

Who's most at risk?
People with high blood pressure, heart disease, lung disease or **kidney disease** (I made that bolded.) are most vulnerable to the effects of humid conditions, as are those over age 50. Other risk factors that can affect your body's ability to cool itself include being obese; having poor circulation; following a salt-restricted diet; drinking alcohol; having inefficient sweat glands; and taking diuretics, sedatives, tranquilizers or heart or blood pressure medication."

So, pretty much, the way to deal with heat and humidity having an effect on your (and my) CKD is to avoid it. That doesn't mean you have to move, you know. Staying in air conditioning as long as you can so your body is not overheated and can better handle this kind of weather will help. Wearing a hat and cool clothes will also help. I certainly relearned the value of wearing cotton this past week. It's a fabric that breathes. I'll bet that this is how those CKD patients who live in humid areas deal with it.

9/4/17 *A Laboring Electrolyte*

It's Labor Day here in the United States. I feel a special affinity for this holiday and wanted to explain the day some more. Oh, I already did in **SlowItDownCKD 2016**:

"For those of you in the United States, here's hoping you have a healthy, safe Labor Day. I come from a union family. So much so that my maternal grandfather was in and out of jail for attempting to unionize brass workers. That was quite a bit of pressure on my grandmother, who raised the four children and ran a restaurant aimed at the men who were saving up funds to bring their families here from Europe. I knew there was more than my personal history with the holiday so I poked around and found this from http://www.usatoday.com/story/news/nation/2016/09/04/labor-day-history/89826440/

'In the late 1800s, the state of labor was grim as U.S. workers toiled under bleak conditions: 12 or more hour workdays; hazardous work environments; meager pay. Children, some as young as 5, were often fixtures at plants and factories. The dismal livelihoods fueled the formation of the country's first labor unions, which began to organize strikes and protests and pushed employers for better hours and pay. Many of the rallies turned violent. On Sept. 5, 1882 — a Tuesday — 10,000 workers took unpaid time off to march in a parade from City Hall to Union Square in New York City as a tribute to American workers. Organized by New York's Central Labor Union, It was the country's first unofficial Labor Day parade. Three years later, some city ordinances marked the first government recognition, and legislation soon followed in a number of states.'"

Now, how do I transition from Labor Day to magnesium? Hmmm, my hard working daughter brought up the subject in today's phone conversation, but that doesn't seem like a good transition.

Aha! Magnesium is a hard working electrolyte. Okay, that works for me.

Let's start off with the basics. This passage from *What Is It and How Did I Get It? Early Stage Chronic Kidney Disease* will give you an idea of what magnesium is and what it may have to do with you as a CKD patient:

"In order to fully understand the renal diet, you need to know a little something about electrolytes. There are the sodium, potassium, and phosphate you've been told about and also calcium, magnesium, chloride and bicarbonate. They maintain balance in your body. This is not the kind of balance that helps you stand upright, but the kind that keeps your body healthy. Too much or too little of a certain electrolyte presents different problems."

Problems? With magnesium? Maybe we need to know what magnesium does for us. The medical dictionary part of The Free Dictionary by Farlex at http://medical-dictionary.thefreedictionary.com/magnesium tells us:

"An alkaline earth element (atomic number 12; atomic weight 24.3) which is an essential mineral required for bone and tooth formation, nerve conduction and muscle contraction; it is required by many enzymes involved in carbohydrate, protein and nucleic acid metabolism. Magnesium is present in almonds, apples, dairy products, corn, figs, fresh leafy greens, legumes, nuts, seafood, seeds, soybeans, wheat germ and whole grains. Magnesium may be useful in treating anxiety, asthma and cardiovascular disease; it is thought to prevent blood clots, raise HDL-cholesterol, lower LDL-cholesterol, reduce arrhythmias and blood pressure, and to help with depression, fatigue, hyperactivity and migraines."

All this by an electrolyte that constitutes only 1% of extra cellular fluid? I'm beginning to suspect that magnesium is the under explained electrolyte. All right then, what happens if you have too little magnesium? Keep in mind that as CKD patients, electrolytes are not being as effectively eliminated by our kidneys as they could be since we have some degree of decline in our kidney function.

The U.S. Dept. of Health & Human Services of the National Institutes of Health at https://ods.od.nih.gov/factsheets/Magnesium-HealthProfessional/ lays it out for us:

"Early signs of magnesium deficiency include loss of appetite, nausea, vomiting, fatigue, and weakness. As magnesium deficiency worsens, numbness, tingling, muscle contractions and cramps, seizures, personality changes, abnormal heart rhythms, and coronary spasms can occur …. Severe magnesium deficiency can result in hypocalcemia or hypokalemia (low serum calcium or potassium levels, respectively) because mineral homeostasis is disrupted…."

Well, who's at risk for magnesium deficiency? The same source tells us:

"Magnesium inadequacy can occur when intakes fall below the RDA but are above the amount required to prevent overt deficiency. The following groups are more likely than others to be at risk of magnesium inadequacy because they typically consume insufficient amounts or they have medical conditions (or take medications) that reduce magnesium absorption from the gut or increase losses from the body.

People with gastrointestinal diseases
The chronic diarrhea and fat malabsorption resulting from Crohn's disease, gluten-sensitive enteropathy (celiac disease), and regional enteritis can lead to magnesium depletion over time …. Resection or bypass of the small intestine, especially the ileum, typically leads to malabsorption and magnesium loss ….

People with type 2 diabetes
Magnesium deficits and increased urinary magnesium excretion can occur in people with insulin resistance and/or type 2 diabetes…. The magnesium loss appears to be secondary to higher concentrations of glucose in the kidney that increase urine output …. People with alcohol dependence
Magnesium deficiency is common in people with chronic alcoholism…. In these individuals, poor dietary intake and nutritional status; gastrointestinal problems, including vomiting, diarrhea, and steatorrhea (fatty stools) resulting from pancreatitis; renal dysfunction with excess excretion of magnesium into the urine; phosphate depletion; vitamin D deficiency; acute alcoholic ketoacidosis; and hyperaldosteronism secondary to liver disease can all contribute to decreased magnesium status ….

Older adults
Older adults have lower dietary intakes of magnesium than younger adults …. In addition, magnesium absorption from the gut decreases and renal magnesium excretion increases with age …. Older adults are also more likely to have chronic diseases or take medications that alter magnesium status, which can increase their risk of magnesium depletion …."

Notice how many times the kidneys were mentioned. Quick, go check your lab results. You'll notice there's no magnesium level. If you'd like your magnesium tested, you or your doctor need to order a specific test for that. Some labs will allow you to order your own magnesium test; others will require a doctor's orders.

9/11/17 *This Former Hippy Wannabe Likes HIPAA*

Each day, I post a tidbit about, or relating to, Chronic Kidney Disease on **SlowItDownCKD's Facebook page**. This is the quote from *Renal and Urology News* that I posted just a short while ago:

"Patients with stage 3 and 4 chronic kidney disease (CKD) who were managed by nephrology in addition to primary care experienced greater monitoring for progression and complications, according to a new study."

My primary care physician is the one who caught my CKD in the first place and is very careful about monitoring its progress. My nephrologist is pleased with that and feels he only needs to see me once a year. The two of them work together well.

From the comments on that post, I realized this is not usual. One of my readers suggested it had to do with HIPPA, so I decided to look into that.

The California Department of Health Care Services (Weird, I know, but I liked their simple explanation.) at http://www.dhcs.ca.gov/formsandpubs/laws/hipaa/Pages/1.00WhatisHIPAA.aspx defined HIPPA and its purposes in the following way:

"HIPAA is the acronym for the Health Insurance Portability and Accountability Act that was passed by Congress in 1996. HIPAA does the following:
• Provides the ability to transfer and continue health insurance coverage for millions of American workers and their families when they change or lose their jobs;
• Reduces health care fraud and abuse;
• Mandates industry-wide standards for health care information on electronic billing and other processes; and

• Requires the protection and confidential handling of protected health information"

Got it. Let's take a look at its last purpose. There is an infogram from HealthIT.gov which greatly clarifies the issue. One item on that infogram caught my eye:

"You hold the key to your health information and can send or have it sent to anyone you want. Only send your health information to someone you trust."

I always send mine to one of my daughters and Bear... and my other doctors if they are not part of the hospital system most of my doctors belong to.

I stumbled across National Conference of State Legislatures at http://www.ncsl.org/research/health/hipaa-a-state-related-overview.aspx and learned more than I even knew existed about HIPAA. Take a look if you'd like more information. I finally tore myself away from the site to get back to writing the blog after following links for about an hour. It was fascinating, but not germane to today's blog.

Okay, so sharing. In order to share the information from one doctor that my other doctors may not have, I simply fill out an Authorization to Release Medical Information form. A copy of this is kept in the originating doctor's files. By the way, it is legal for the originating doctor to charge $.75/page for each page sent, but none of my doctors have ever done so.

I know, I know. What is this about doctors being part of the hospital system? What hospital system? When I first looked for a new physician since the one I had been using was so far away (Over the usual half-an-hour-to-get-anywhere-in-Arizona rule), I saw that my new PCP's practice was affiliated with the local hospital and thought nothing of it.

Then Electronic Health Records came into widespread use at this hospital. Boom! Any doctor associated with that hospital – and that's all but two of my myriad doctors – instantly had access to my health records. Wow, no more requesting hard copies of my health records from each doctor, making copies for all my other doctors, and then hand delivering or mailing them. No wonder I'm getting lazy; life is so much easier.

Back to HealthIt.gov for more about EHR. This time at https://www.healthit.gov/buzz-blog/electronic-health-and-medical-records/emr-vs-ehr-difference/:

"With fully functional EHRs, all members of the team have ready access to the latest information allowing for more coordinated, patient-centered care. With EHRs:
• The information gathered by the primary care provider tells the emergency department clinician about the patient's life threatening allergy, so that care can be adjusted appropriately, even if the patient is unconscious.
• A patient can log on to his own record and see the trend of the lab results over the last year, which can help motivate him to take his medications and keep up with the lifestyle changes that have improved the numbers.
• The lab results run last week are already in the record to tell the specialist what she needs to know without running duplicate tests.
• The clinician's notes from the patient's hospital stay can help inform the discharge instructions and follow-up care and enable the patient to move from one care setting to another more smoothly."

Did you notice the part about what a patient can do? With my patient portal, I can check my labs, ask questions, schedule an appointment, obtain information about medications, and spot trends in my labs.

Lazy? Let's make that even lazier. No more appointments for trivial questions, no more leaving phone messages, no more being on hold for too long. I find my care is quicker, more accessible to me, and – believe it or not – more easily understood since I am a visual, rather than an audial, person.

9/18/17 *Memories of Another Sort*

When I was teaching Creative Non-Fiction at Phoenix College, I got into the habit of taking my classes to The Poisoned Pen, an award winning independent book store here in Arizona. I wanted them to hear well known authors talk about their writing process and see that these people were human beings just as they, my students, were. I retired from teaching several years ago, but I still go to writers' workshops at the Pen. Last time I was there, I stumbled upon an advance copy of a book by Lisa Stone.

What's an advance copy? It means either Advance Reading Copy of Advance Review Copy – depending upon who you talk to and is abbreviated ARC. TCK Publishing at https://www.tckpublishing.com/advance-review-copies/ informs us:

"Big traditional publishers often print thousands of ARC copies to send out to trade reviewers, bloggers, booksellers, librarians, and other people who can generate word of mouth for the book. In today's technological environment, digital ARCs are gaining rapidly in popularity, sent out in email blasts and through various online services. ARCs are also used in giveaways and contests to give ordinary readers early access to books in an effort to build buzz."

Lisa Stone, the author of the ARC of *The Darkness Within* (the one I picked up), is the nom de plume of Kathy Glass. She's a bestselling British author who wrote about cellular memory – alternately called cellular memory phenomenon – after organ transplant. I was transfixed.

We all know I rarely write about transplantation, but today I am. Here's a reminder from *SlowItDownCKD 2015* as to just what that is:

"WebMD at http://www.webmd.com/a-to-z-guides/kidney-transplant-20666 tells us:

'A kidney transplant is surgery to replace your own diseased kidneys with a healthy (donor) kidney.'

I should mention that while there are transplants from both living and cadaver donors, both will require lifelong drugs to prevent rejection. "

Now for the biggie: what is cellular memory? According to Medical Daily at http://www.medicaldaily.com/can-organ-transplant-change-recipients-personality-cell-memory-theory-affirms-yes-247498:

"The behaviors and emotions acquired by the recipient from the original donor are due to the combinatorial memories stored in the neurons of the organ donated. Heart transplants are said to be the most susceptible to cell memory where organ transplant recipients experienced a change of heart."

Lisa Stone's protagonist had a heart transplant and his personality became that of his donor. Far fetched? Maybe.

But what about the case of Demi-Lee Brennan, the Australian young lady who had a liver transplant that changed her blood type and immune system back in 2008? The Sydney Morning Herald at http://www.smh.com.au/news/national/transplant-girls-blood-change-a-miracle/2008/01/24/1201157559928.html included this quote from one of her doctors.

"'We didn't believe this at first. We thought it was too strange to be true,' Dr Alexander said. 'Normally the body's own immune system rejects any cells that are transplanted ... but for some reason the cells that came from the donor's liver seemed to survive better than Demi-Lee's own cells. It has huge implications for the future of organ transplants.'"

And those who have received kidney transplants? Is there anything to report about cellular memory there? I turned to the Daily Mail, a British newspaper, at http://www.dailymail.co.uk/health/article-533830/My-personality-changed-kidney-transplant–I-started-read-Jane-Austen-Dostoevsky-instead-celebrity-trash.html#ixzz4t3Ml4sAt and found this:

"'A spokesman for UK Transplant said: 'While we are aware of the suggestion that transplant recipients take on aspects of the personality of the organ donor, we are not aware of any evidence to support it.

While not discarding it entirely, we have no reason to believe that it happens. We would be interested to see any definitive evidence that supports it.'

Examples cited as proof of cellular memory include a U.S. woman terrified of heights who became a climber and a seven-year-old girl who had nightmares about being killed after being given the heart of a murdered child."

The Liberty Voice, a publication that is new to me and seems to be part of The Guardian, at http://guardianlv.com/2013/06/organ-transplants-cellular-memory-proves-major-organs-have-self-contained-brains/ had the sort of background information I was looking for:

"In our modern culture, cellular memory was first studied in heart transplant recipients when the patients displayed strange cravings, change in tastes, cravings and mild personality. Major organs like the heart, liver, kidney, and even muscles are known to contain large populations of neural networks, which are self-contained brains and produce noticeable changes. Acquired combinatorial memories in organ transplants could enable transferred organs to respond to patterns familiar to the organ donors, and it may be triggered by emotional signals. Science discovered evidence that nervous system organs store memories and respond to places, events, and people recognized by their donors.

Gary Schwartz has documented the cases of 74 patients, 23 of whom were heart transplant recipients. Transfers of memories have not been reported in simpler transplants like corneas because they don't contain large population of neurons. Dr. Andrew Armour a pioneer in neurocardiology suggests that the brain has two-way communication links with the 'little brain in the heart.' The intelligence of neural brains in organs depends on memories stored in nerve cells."

Since I didn't know the publication, I checked on some of the contributors...especially since the documentation was on such a small population. Well, will you look at that; Gary Schwartz is a local teaching at The University of Arizona. This is his faculty entry in the Department of Neurology.

"Dr. Schwartz is Professor of Psychology, Medicine, Neurology, Psychiatry and Surgery. He is the Director of the Laboratory for Advances in Consciousness and Health (LACH, formerly the Human Energy Systems Laboratory). After receiving his doctorate from Harvard University, he served as a professor of psychology and psychiatry at Yale University, director of the Yale Psychophysiology Center, and co-director of the Yale Behavioral Medicine Clinic. Dr. Schwartz has published more than four hundred scientific papers, edited eleven academic books, is the author of several books including The Afterlife Experiments, The Truth About Medium, The G.O.D. Experiments, and The Energy Healing Experiments."

9/25/17 *Feed Me*

Over the years, I've seen advertisements for food preparation services. You know the ones that cook your meals and deliver them weekly. I would approach the people offering the service to see what they could do with the renal diet. That was a deal killer right there.

All right, I figured. Maybe what I should be doing is finding a chef who is willing to work with kidney patients rather than asking existing food preparation services to accommodate just me. I even had one chef who agreed that this is a valuable service and something she wanted to do. I was excited. Then she simply stopped emailing and answering calls. That was a couple of years ago.
I sort of gave up... until I ran into an advertisement for Clarence's food service. I figured it was worth it to try again and called him. It was.

I explained to Clarence that I don't permit advertising on my blog, but I would like other Chronic Kidney Disease patients to see how they can make use of food preparation services such as his. He was kind enough to write this guest blog for us. I'm hoping that this inspires you to approach a chef in your area to ask him/her if he/she is willing to provide such a service. Of course, not all of us want to have someone else prepare our meals or want to spend the money to do so, so this is a blog for that portion of readers who do.

Meal Planning for Those with Kidney Disease.
Clarence Ferguson, RTSM, CMTA, NT

Understanding your kidney disease, or renal disease, is the first step in taking control of your health. While I am not a doctor, I have aligned myself with those whose specialize in CKD so that I can adjust meals accordingly. When you have kidney disease, your kidneys are no longer able to remove waste effectively from your body or to balance your fluids. The buildup of wastes can change the chemistry of your body causing some symptoms that you can feel, and others that you don't.

With kidney diseases, the first symptoms you may have are ones that you won't feel but that will show up in tests that your doctor orders. Common problems are high blood pressure, anemia and weakening bones. It is important to find a kidney doctor (also called a nephrologist). And once you have your doctor's recommendation that's where we come in and prepare your meal according to his or her recommendations.

Okay Clarence, we know that but how do we navigate healthy eating?

Here are some suggestions for you and what I prepare for clients who struggle with CKD.

Make sure these snacks are readily available:
1. Fruit: apples, grapes, tangerines or strawberries; dried cranberries or blueberries; or packaged fruit cups with diced peaches, pears, pineapple, mandarin oranges or mixed fruit. Make sure they are organic.
2. Low- or no-sodium microwave popcorn.
3. Low-sodium crackers, pita chips or unsalted pretzels.
4. Pouches of tuna or chicken and a side of Vegainse (a dairy free option for mayonnaise).
5. Kidney-friendly nutrition bars or liquid supplements, such as the ones from ID life, since they meet these guidelines.

What we do at Fit Body Foods
1. Compare brands. Sodium and potassium levels can vary significantly from one brand to another.
2. Look for low-sodium labels on packaging. Stock up on the low-

est sodium broths, stocks and condiments.
3. Choose fresh vegetables, or frozen or canned veggies with no added salt or sodium.
4. Use only 1/4 as much of the tomato sauce and canned tomatoes that a recipe calls for to limit potassium and sodium.
5. Don't use canned fish or chicken with added salt. All fish is fresh, so we can control the sodium levels by rinsing to reduce the sodium. Try to limit use of canned goods in general.
6. Avoid baking and pancake mixes that have salt and baking powder added. Instead, make a kidney-friendly recipe from scratch.
7. Use sweet pickles instead of dill pickles and check for added salt.
8. Check cold and instant hot cereals for sodium amounts. Although oatmeal contains more phosphorus than some cereals, it may be okay one to two times a week if phosphorus is well-controlled.
9. Check the ingredients in vinegar. Some vinegars, such as seasoned rice vinegar, contain added salt and sugar.
10. Avoid store-bought sauces and gravies that have mystery ingredients in them. Make our own instead from real-food ingredients.
11. Use homemade soup recipes, such as Rotisserie Chicken Noodle Soup, instead of pre-made or canned soups. Some soups contain more than 800 mg sodium per serving.
12. Low – and reduced – sodium broth is great for use in cooking. We save the homemade broth from stewed or boiled chicken or beef.
13. Don't trade sodium for potassium. Some products replace salt with potassium chloride.
14. Limit nuts, seeds and chocolate as they are high in potassium and phosphorus.

We prepare food weekly and deliver to our clients on Sundays. We take the worry out of meal prep, our meals start at $7.99 a meal, and we can accommodate most palates. We can be reached for orders at: info@coachclarence.com.

Below is a sample recipe:

Cucumber-Carrot Salad
Diet types: CKD non-dialysis, Dialysis, Diabetes
Portions: 4
Serving size: 1/2 cup
Ingredients:
1/4 cup unseasoned rice vinegar
1 teaspoon sugar
1/2 teaspoon olive oil
1/8 teaspoon black pepper
1/2 cucumber
1 cup carrots
2 tablespoons green onion
2 tablespoons red bell pepper
1/2 teaspoon Mrs. Dash® Italian Medley seasoning blend

Notice there is nothing new here. We all know this information. What is appealing is having someone else, someone who understands our diet limitations, buy the food and prepare it for our meals. I explained to Clarence that our food needs as far as electrolytes change with each blood test and he agreed that it's important to eat according to your numbers. That's something he's very willing to pay attention to. Should this interest you, why not approach a professional in your area to see if they can also provide such a service?

10/2/17 *Helping Where You Can*

When my brothers made it public that they each had Parkinson's' Disease several years ago, I decided to see how I could help. They were being well taken care of by their wives and their medical teams, so they didn't need my help. Maybe I could help others, I reasoned. So I began exploring ways I might be able to do that... and found one.

It was clear clinical trials with people of my heritage were being conducted and needed participants. It wasn't clear what these studies entailed. They weren't reader friendly enough for me to understand, but after multiple emails and phone calls asking for clarification, I finally understood. During the whole process, I kept thinking to myself that this was a wonderful way to help if only it were more accessible – meaning more easily understood.

A couple of weeks ago, *Antidote Match* approached me about carrying their widget on my blog roll. If you look at the lists on the right side of the blog, you'll see it in turquoise. Actually, I chose turquoise because you just can't miss that color.

According to the National Institutes of Health (part of the U.S. Department of Health and Human Services) at https://www.nhlbi.nih.gov/studies/clinicaltrials/ :

"Clinical trials are research studies that explore whether a medical strategy, treatment, or device is safe and effective for humans. These studies also may show which medical approaches work best for certain illnesses or groups of people. Clinical trials produce the best data available for health care decision making.

The purpose of clinical trials is research, so the studies follow strict scientific standards. These standards protect patients and help produce reliable study results.

Clinical trials are one of the final stages of a long and careful re-search process. The process often begins in a laboratory (lab), where scientists first develop and test new ideas.

If an approach seems promising, the next step may involve animal testing. This shows how the approach affects a living body and whether it's harmful. However, an approach that works well in the lab or animals doesn't always work well in people. Thus, research in humans is needed.

For safety purposes, clinical trials start with small groups of pa-tients to find out whether a new approach causes any harm. In later phases of clinical trials, researchers learn more about the new approach's risks and benefits.

A clinical trial may find that a new strategy, treatment, or device
• improves patient outcomes;
• offers no benefit; or
• causes unexpected harm

All of these results are important because they advance medical knowledge and help improve patient care".

Important, right? But why *Antidote Match*, you ask? That's easy: because it's easy. The information offered is in lay language, the common language you and I understand, rather than in medi-calese. Maybe I should just let them present their own case:

"Antidote Match™

Matching patients to trials in a completely new way
Antidote Match is the world's smartest clinical trial matching tool, allowing patients to match to trials just by answering a few ques-tions about their health.

Putting technology to work
We have taken on the massive job of structuring all publicly available clinical trial eligibility criteria so that it is machine-readable and searchable. This means that for the first time, through a machine-learning algorithm that dynamically selects questions, patients can answer just a few questions to search through thousands of trials within a given therapeutic area in seconds and find one that's right for them. Patients receive trial information that is specific to their condition with clear contact information to get in touch with researchers.

Reaching patients where they are
Even the smartest search tool is only as good as the number of people who use it, so we've made our search tool available free of charge to patient communities, advocacy groups, and health portals. We're proud to power clinical trial search on more than a hundred of these sites, reaching millions of patients per month where they are already looking for health information.

Translating scientific jargon
Our platform pulls information on all the trials listed on clinicaltrials.gov and presents it into a simple, patient-friendly design.
You (Gail here: this point is addressed to the ones conducting the clinical trial) then have the option to augment that content through our free tool, Antidote Bridge™, to include the details that are most important to patients – things like number of overnights, compensation, and procedures used. This additional information helps close the information gap between patients and researchers, which ultimately yields greater engagement with patients.

Here's how Antidote Match works
1. Visit search engine → Patients visit either our website or one of the sites that host our search.
2. Enter condition → They enter the condition in which they're

interested, and begin answering the questions as they appear
3. Answer questions → As more questions are answered, the number of clinical trial matches reduces
4. Get in touch: When they're ready, patients review their matches and can get in touch with the researchers running each study directly through our tool

A bit about Antidote
Antidote is a digital health company on a mission to accelerate the breakthroughs of new treatments by bridging the gap between medical research and the people who need them. We have commercial agreements with the majority of the top 25 pharmaceutical companies and CROs, and a partner network that is growing every day.

Antidote was launched as TrialReach in 2010 and rebranded to Antidote in 2016. We're based in New York, NY and London, U.K. For more information, visit www.antidote.me ...."

Try it from the blog roll. I did. I was going to include my results, but realized they wouldn't be helpful since my address, age, sex, diseases, and conditions may be different from everyone else's. One caveat: search for Chronic Renal Insufficiency or Chronic Renal Failure (whichever applies to you) rather than Chronic Kidney Disease.

10/9/17 *Book It!*

Every once in a great while, I'll come across a Chronic Kidney Disease book that I want to share. I think there were only three or four of these in the last six years. Today, I add another one. Dr. Kang, the author, is a local doctor. That was the first thing that caught my eye.

I thought I would be reading the usual information … and I did, but it was written with verve and included some information I hadn't known. So I did the obvious. I contacted the good doctor to see if he'd be interested in sharing his knowledge with us on the blog. I'm so very glad he agreed.

Dr. Mandip S.Kang, is not only a senior partner in Southwest Kidney Institute right here in Phoenix, but he is also a Fellow in the American Society of Nephrologists I like so much. I often refer to them in both my blogs and books. He is also the author of the IBPA Gold Award winning book: *The Doctor's Kidney Diets……A Nutritional Guide to Managing and Slowing The Progression of Chronic Kidney Disease*, the book that caught my eye.

This is what he wrote for us:

"Receiving a diagnosis of kidney disease is not a death sentence for patients, but is often overwhelming and a life changing event. Patients are often confused and the information they receive from different healthcare providers may not be the same. Patients often ask, 'What should I do?'

Having experience as a former Assistant Clinical Professor of Medicine at University of Utah School of Medicine and currently as a Senior Nephrologist (kidney specialist), I have gained some insight into how to alleviate my patients' fears and I have come up with a four point plan that I try to teach my kidney patients. I believe that the role of the physician is to be a teacher and a coach as patients navigate their way into the complexities of a Chronic Kidney Disease diagnosis. I believe that every kidney specialist should have a chalk board in the patient exam rooms and lay out the plan for his or her approach to their patients just like we were taught in schools.

Here is a four point plan that all kidney patients should remember as they visit their kidney specialists and at home. The acronym for the plan is very simple: D.A.M.E.

1. 'D' in the acronym stands for diet. The reason I chose diet first comes from the Chinese wisdom in treating any disease: 'He that takes medicine and neglects diet, wastes the skills of the physician.' Patients must be taught what the kidney diet is and why they need to follow it for the rest of their lives. Since the kidney diet is complex, they must be provided with educational materials that outline the diet and be strongly encouraged to visit a kidney dietitian who will tell them what and how much to eat. Dietitians and kidney doctors will teach them about the benefits of eating fresh foods and avoiding processed foods. Patients should remember that the 'p' in 'p'rocessed foods is akin to 'p'acked with calories. Learning to read a Nutrition Facts label is a must if the doctor wants to do all he or she can to help the patient slow down – and sometimes halt – the progression of kidney disease. It is important to remember that in the earlier stages of kidney disease, the diet may not be as strict – but if progression of the disease is noted, then dietary modifications are more stringent and frequent laboratory tests may need to be performed to assess progress.

2. 'A' in the four point CKD plan stands for activity. "What is activity?" you might say. It could mean walking more, taking more steps daily, joining a gym, hiking, biking or any activity that keeps you on your feet. As most Americans already know, the obesity rates in

the USA are skyrocketing leading to most chronic health conditions such as Chronic Kidney Disease, Coronary Artery Disease, Stroke, Arthritis, Lung Disease, etc. These chronic health conditions stem from lack of activity and consuming excessive calories. Many patients lead a sedentary lifestyle such as watching TV for long hours which leads to worsening of their health issues. Patients should be encouraged to do the activities they enjoy the most such as dancing, or walking in a park or on a beach. Patients should weigh themselves on a weekly basis to monitor their weight.

3. 'M' in the acronym stands for medications that your doctor prescribes. Your doctor may also tell you not to take certain over the counter medications that may harm your kidneys such as Advil, Motrin, Aleve, Ibuprofen, Celebrex, Prilosec, herbal remedies, etc. I encourage all patients to memorize their medications and keep a list with them at all times. Remember that all medications are prescribed because the benefit to the patient outweighs the risk and no medication is entirely safe; therefore, it should be taken as prescribed and any side effects reported to your doctor. You should not take any new medicine unless it has been cleared by your kidney specialist.

4. 'E' in the above acronym stands for education. This is the key element in the D.A.M.E plan to treat patients with CKD. Unless the patient has a clear understanding of their disease process, labs, treatment plan, and the role of diet, activity, and medications, they will not be successful in managing and slowing the progression of Chronic Kidney Disease. How well a patient does will depend on their knowledge of their disease and if they comply with the instructions given to them by the kidney doctors.
I hope that all kidney doctors and patients keep the D.A.M.E. acronym in mind. Patients who are active participants in their care lead healthier and productive lives. I wish all of the readers well."

I hadn't heard of the D.A.M.E. method before but I like it, especially "the 'p' in 'p'rocessed foods is akin to 'p'acked with calories." Many thanks, Dr. Kang, for introducing this common sense theme to us.

10/16/17 *Sex?*

I know, I know. When you see that question on an application, you want to answer 'yes,' but you're only given the choice of male or female. Well, at least that's my experience. Okay, got that out of the way.

Way back in 2011, the following was included in my first Chronic Kidney Disease book, *What Is It and How Did I Get It? Early Stage Chronic Kidney Disease*. This was way before the website, Facebook page, blog, Instagram, Pinterest, Twitter, and LinkedIn accounts. Way before the articles, radio shows, and interviews, book signings, and talks about CKD. Come to think of it, this was way before *SlowItDownCKD* was born.

"I haven't found too much about sex that's different from the problems of non-CKD patients although with this disease there may be a lower sex drive accompanied by a loss of libido and an inability to ejaculate. Usually, these problems start with an inability to keep an erection as long as usual. The resulting impotency has a valid physical, psychological or psycho-physical cause.

Some of the physical causes of impotence, more recently referred to as Erectile Dysfunction [E.D.] for a CKD patient could be poor blood supply since there are narrowed blood vessels all over the body. Or maybe it's leaky blood vessels. Of course, it could be a hormonal disturbance since the testicles may be producing less testosterone and the kidneys are in charge of hormones....

While E.D. can be caused by renal disease, it can also be caused by diabetes and hypertension. All three are of importance to CKD patients. Sometimes, E.D. is caused by the medications for hypertension, depression and anxiety. But, E.D. can also be caused by other diseases, injuries, surgeries, prostate cancer or a host of other conditions and bodily malfunctions. Psychologically, the problem may be caused by stress, low self-esteem, even guilt to name just a few of the possible causes….

Women with CKD may also suffer from sexual problems, but the causes can be complicated. As with men, renal disease, diabetes and hypertension may contribute to the problem. But so can poor body image, low self-esteem, depression, stress and sexual abuse. Any chronic disease can make a man or a woman feel less sexual….

Common sense tells us that sex or intimacy is not high on your list of priorities when you've just been recently diagnosed…. Sometimes people with chronic diseases can be so busy being the patient that they forget their partners have needs, too. And sometimes, remembering to stay close, really close as in hugging and snuggling, can be helpful…".

Well, what's changed since I was writing *What Is It and How Did I Get It? Early Stage Chronic Kidney Disease?* in 2010?

The National Kidney Foundation at https://www.kidney.org/atoz/content/sexuality now includes the following on their website:

"It's important to remember that people with kidney failure can have healthy marriages and meaningful relationships. They can fall in love, care for families, and be sexual. Staying intimate with those you love is important. It's something everyone needs.

Many people think that sexuality refers only to sexual intercourse. But sexuality includes many things, like touching, hugging, or kissing. It includes how you feel about yourself, how well you communicate, and how willing you are to be close to someone else. There are many things that can affect your sexuality if you have kidney disease or kidney failure — hormones, nerves, energy levels, even medicine. But there are also things you and your healthcare team can do to deal with these changes. Don't be afraid to ask questions or get help from a healthcare professional."

DaVita at https://www.davita.com/kidney-disease/overview/living-with-ckd/sexuality-and-chronic-kidney-disease/e/4895 also offers advice:

"Once again, it's important to remember, you are not alone. There are no limits with regard to sexual activities you may engage in as a patient with renal disease, as long as activity does not place pressure or tension on the access site, causing damage. (Me: This is for advanced CKD.)

If you are sexually active, practicing safe sex and/or using birth control are needed, even if you think you may be physically unable to have children.

Activities such as touching, hugging and kissing provide feelings of warmth and closeness even if intercourse is not involved. Professional sex therapists can recommend alternative methods as well. Keeping an open mind and having a positive attitude about yourself and your sexuality may lower the chances of having sexual problems.

There are both medical and emotional causes for sexual dysfunction. The reason for your dysfunction can be determined through a thorough physical exam in addition to an assessment of your emotional welfare and coping skills.

Relaxation techniques, physical exercise, writing in a journal and talking to your social worker or a therapist can help you to feel better about your body image and/or sexual dysfunction. Resuming previous activities, such as dining out or traveling, as a couple or single adult, can be helpful.

Provide tokens of affection or simple acts of kindness to show you care.

Communicate with your partner or others about how you feel." According to the Kidney Foundation of Canada, these may be the causes of sexual problems in CKD.

"Fatigue is a major factor. Any chronic illness is tiring, and chronic kidney disease, which is often accompanied by anemia and a demanding treatment, practically guarantees fatigue.

Depression is another common issue. Almost everyone experiences periods of depression, and one of the symptoms of depression is loss of interest in sexual intimacy.

Medications can also affect one's ability or desire to have intercourse. Since there may be other medications which are just as effective without the side effect of loss of sexual function or desire, talk to your doctor about your pills.

Feelings about body image (Having a peritoneal catheter, or a fistula or graft), may cause some people to avoid physical contact for fear of feeling less attractive or worrying about what people think when they look at them. (Me: Again, this is for late stage CKD.) Some diseases, such as vascular disease and diabetes, can lead to decreased blood flow in the genital area, decreased sexual desire, vaginal dryness and impotence."

It looks like the information about CKD and sexuality hasn't changed that much, but it does seem to be more available these days.

10/23/17 *Not a Drug, a Medical Food*

On a Facebook Chronic Kidney Disease support page, I mentioned that I use a medical food to help with my osteoarthritis. And then the questions started flying. Those of us who would prefer no more Rx drugs seemed the most interested. I already take Rx drugs for both hyperlipidemia and hypertension. I didn't want to add yet another Rx drug that may have side effects. This is a lot safer for my poor little kidneys.

Let's start at the beginning with a definition. According to the Free Dictionary's Medical Dictionary at http://medical-dictionary.thefreedictionary.com/Medical+food, a medical food is:

"A food formulated by the selective use of nutrients and manufactured for the dietary treatment of a specific condition or disease."

I am not referring to dietary supplements here, but rather a replacement for a drug that can be prescribed for a specific disease. In my case, it's osteoarthritis. CoverMyMedicalFoods.com explains that:

"Medical foods are prescription medicines made from natural molecules found in food. One pill can equal natural ingredients found in five pounds of fruits and vegetables. Purified, natural ingredients equal fewer side effects. Large amounts of these purified molecules help the body fight disease.

Unlike dietary supplements or Rx drugs, the ingredients are designated G.R.A.S. 'Generally Recognized as Safe,' which is the highest standard of safety at the FDA. Also unlike dietary supplements or Rx drugs, medical foods are intended for a disease or condition that has distinctive nutritional requirements.

Like Rx drugs, but unlike dietary supplements, they must be supervised by a physician and dispensed by prescription. (My rheumatologist performs this task for me.)"

Pharmacist Gayle Nicholas Scott explains The Federal Food and Drug Administration's (FDA) rules for medical foods on Medscape.

"The FDA specifies that medical foods are foods specifically formulated for dietary management of diseases or conditions with distinctive nutritional needs that cannot be met by diet alone. Generally, a product must meet the following criteria to be labeled a 'medical food':

• A specific formulation (as opposed to a naturally occurring foodstuff in its natural state) for oral or tube feeding;
• Labeled for the dietary management of a specific medical disorder, disease, or condition with distinctive nutritional requirements;
• Intended for use under medical supervision; and
• Intended only for a patient receiving active and ongoing medical supervision for a condition requiring medical care on a recurring basis so that instructions on the use of the medical food can be provided."

This was all getting a bit technical so I decided to go to my medical food's website for an example. I take Limbrel. This is from their website.

"Limbrel is a prescription medical food product for the daily nutritional management of the metabolic aspects of osteoarthritis. Limbrel is not a drug, nor a dietary supplement. Because Limbrel is a Medical Food (MF) product, we are required to describe it differently from how a drug or dietary supplement is described.

By statutory and regulatory definition, product claims must be explicitly different for medical food products versus drugs versus dietary supplements. Generally, Medical Food claims reference the 'dietary management' or 'distinctive nutritional requirements' of a particular disease or the metabolic processes of that disease, whereas drug claims reference 'curing, treating, preventing or mitigating' the effects or symptoms of a particular disease, while dietary supplement claims reference 'supporting' healthy function of the body or particular body organ or system.

First, osteoarthritis patients are shown to have distinctive nutritional requirements and metabolic imbalances. Then, for example, a Medical Food may claim the dietary management of metabolic processes of osteoarthritis, whereas a drug may claim the reduction of osteoarthritis pain, while a dietary supplement may claim the support of overall health of joints. A Medical Food must meet the distinctive nutritional requirements of a disease through dietary management, whereas a drug may address the symptoms of a disease or its treatment or prevention of the disease.

Claims for both MFs and drugs must be supported by solid laboratory and clinical data. But, by contrast, for a drug, the safety of the product and both the therapeutic claims and the ingredients must be pre-approved by the FDA through extensive clinical testing. MFs have up-front safety obtained through GRAS (Generally Recognized As Safe) status of the ingredients, including use of the food or food additive or component in perhaps millions of people, whereas drugs have unproven safety that must first be shown in animals and then be tested in human clinical trials, which typically exclude wider populations with various health problems. Medical Food ingredients have GRAS designation, the highest FDA standard of safety given to food. Most MFs are also tested in clinical trials to confirm their 'traditional use' safety.

The use of Medical Food, regulated by the FDA, represents an entirely different approach to managing diseases. For example, unlike drugs, Limbrel does not treat or mask the symptoms of osteoarthritis. Instead, Limbrel manages the underlying metabolic processes of osteoarthritis to restore the proper metabolic balance of inflammatory metabolites at the cellular level, and thereby promotes normal physiologic function."

A little reminder is in order here: metabolic has to do with your metabolism. The Merriam Webster Dictionary at https://www.merriam-webster.com/dictionary/metabolism defines that as

"a: the sum of the processes in the buildup and destruction of protoplasm; specifically: the chemical changes in living cells by which energy is provided for vital processes and activities and new material is assimilated...
• Regular exercise can help to increase your metabolism.
b: the sum of the processes by which a particular substance is handled in the living body
c: the sum of the metabolic activities taking place in a particular environment
• the metabolism of a lake"

I believe it's the second definition that concerns us here.

What I can say for certain is that, at one point, I doubted it was worth the $50 a month to pay for this medical food so I stopped it. That was a mistake. In retrospect, it seemed that my body's reaction to stopping was instantaneous... which I doubt is possible. But my elbows started to hurt too much, so I got my prescription. While I may feel some aches and pains on those rare rainy Arizona days, I am relatively pain free the rest of the time.

10/30/17 *There's Always the Exception*

And this is one of them. We all know I don't write about dialysis, but I've been receiving bunches of emails lately asking if I would consider including this product, that book, or the other social media kidney disease awareness item. My response is usually thank you, but I don't allow advertising or product promotion on the blog. When Dr. Bruce Greenfield, a Los Angeles nephrologist with 37 years experience, sent me a link to his dialysis rap with the following message, I was forced to think twice:

"My goal is to reach every dialysis patient in America, in part to make people more informed, in part to shed a little light into their world in a fun way, and of course- to make them smile!"

But why? Are smiles and laughter necessary in the treatment of illness? According to Dr. Jordan Knox, a resident in family medicine, they are. This is how he summarized the need for physicians to use humor in his essay on KevinMD.com at http://www.kevinmd.com/blog/2017/10/theres-place-humor-medicine.html last Friday:

"Patch Adams, MD is one of the best-known physicians to use humor in healing. He focuses more on silliness to reach pure joy, nourishing the soul as much as the body. There is something about the contrast, when silliness uproots the expectation of seriousness, that is more powerful than pure humor alone. I think that's why humor can be so powerful in the doctor's office; because the expectation is all business, seriousness, and authority. Humor can break down those rigid roles of "patient" and "doctor," or "team leader" and "team member." It can level the playing field and align people on the same side, working toward a shared goal."

Being a Groucho Marx fan, I keep thinking of his one liner, "A clown is like an aspirin, only he works twice as fast."

Hey, CKD patients can't take aspirin (if they're NSAIDS or non-steroidal anti-inflammatory drugs), so why not take humor instead?

But what happens to us physically when we laugh? I checked in with my old standby, The Mayo Clinic, at https://www.mayoclinic.org/healthy-lifestyle/stress-management/in-depth/stress-relief/art-20044456?pg=1 and found the following information about laughter and your body.

"Short-term benefits

Laughter can:
Stimulate many organs. Laughter enhances your intake of oxygen-rich air, stimulates your heart, lungs and muscles, and increases the endorphins that are released by your brain.

Activate and relieve your stress response. A rollicking laugh fires up and then cools down your stress response, and it can increase your heart rate and blood pressure. The result? A good, relaxed feeling.

Soothe tension. Laughter can also stimulate circulation and aid muscle relaxation, both of which can help reduce some of the physical symptoms of stress".

Keep in mind that I am not a dialysis patient but hope that this rap is helpful to those who are. Sit back, turn up the speakers, and have some short term benefits courtesy of Dr. Greenfield.

I laughed… and I learned, but I was really interested in the effects of laughter that could help Chronic Kidney Disease patients in the early and moderate stages. WebMD at https://www.webmd.com/balance/features/give-your-body-boost-with-laughter#2 had a bit more information about that.

Mind you, these results are observational or the results of very small studies.

"Blood flow. Researchers at the University of Maryland studied the effects on blood vessels when people were shown either comedies or dramas. After the screening, the blood vessels of the group who watched the comedy behaved normally — expanding and contracting easily. But the blood vessels in people who watched the drama tended to tense up, restricting blood flow. Immune response. Increased stress is associated with decreased immune system response, says Provine. (He's a professor of psychology and neuroscience at the University of Maryland, Baltimore County and author of Laughter: A Scientific Investigation.) Some studies have shown that the ability to use humor may raise the level of infection-fighting antibodies in the body and boost the levels of immune cells, as well.

Blood sugar levels. One study of 19 people with diabetes looked at the effects of laughter on blood sugar levels. After eating, the group attended a tedious lecture. On the next day, the group ate the same meal and then watched a comedy. After the comedy, the group had lower blood sugar levels than they did after the lecture."

Reminder: Diabetes is the number one cause of CKD. CKD means a compromised immune system. Healthy blood flow is necessary for healthy kidneys.

I don't think we can forget that anything that's good for your heart will benefit the kidneys. Since CKD is an inflammatory disease, reducing inflammation of any kind in the body can only be a good thing. Look at that! Both bad cholesterol and systolic blood will be lowered. These are all kidney related. Hypertension is the second most common cause of CKD. Cholesterol makes the heart work harder, which can raise your blood pressure. Uh-oh.

Another thing I realized is that if I find something wrong, you know like the termite invasion or the a/c breaking in 100 degree weather, my first response is laughter. I never knew why. Hmmm, maybe I've been protecting my body all along.

Obituary

The Book of Blogs: Moderate Stage Chronic Kidney Disease, Part 1 died peacefully on October 20th, 2017, on Amazon.com and B & N.com at the age of three. *The Book of Blogs: Moderate Stage Chronic Kidney Disease, Part 1* is survived by *SlowItDownCKD 2011* & *SlowItDownCKD 2012*, which were both born of a need for larger print, more comprehensive indexes, and a less wieldy book to hold. *The Book of Blogs: Moderate Stage Chronic Kidney Disease, Part 1* was preceded by *What Is It and How Did I Get It? Early Stage Chronic Kidney Disease*. *The Book of Blogs: Moderate Stage Chronic Kidney Disease, Part 1* gave birth to *The Book of Blogs: Moderate Stage Chronic Kidney Disease, Part 2*, *SlowItDownCKD 2015* and *SlowItDownCKD 2016*. Flowers and condolences in the form of Chronic Kidney Disease Awareness may be sent to any and all vehicles for spreading awareness of this disease.

11/6/17 *Snap, Crackle, and Pop*

I haven't taken to eating boxed cereals, although I do thank Rice Krispies for coming up with that slogan. I've discovered there are drawbacks to being independent that I hadn't thought about... like the one that landed me in my new chiropractor's office where I heard those sounds coming from within my body.

It started off so innocently. Our outdoor swing bit the dust so Bear took it apart. I decided our hammock chairs would look great where the swing had been. Ah, but Bear was busy moving the parts of the swing from that part of the patio.

I could do it if I went slowly. So I pulled one of them partway down the walkway, then pulled the second one. Of course, pulling meant going backwards. Why I was looking forward instead of backward, I'll never know. I managed to trip over the foot of the first hammock frame.

My arm was scraped from one end to the other. My thigh had the biggest black and blue mark I'd seen on my body to date. But worse of all, my neck hurt. No problem, I figured. I'll just wash out the scrapes, ice the neck and the thigh and I'll be fine. But I wasn't. Hence, the chiropractic visits.

It's been two weeks. The arm is almost healed, the black and blue mark moving toward disappearing and the neck barely hurts at all. Hmmm, if chiropractic is so good for these aches and pains, could it also be good for my kidneys?

The Medical Dictionary of The Free Dictionary at http://medical-dictionary.thefreedictionary.com/chiropractic defines chiropractic for us:

"Chiropractic is from Greek words meaning done by hand. It is grounded in the principle that the body can heal itself when the skeletal system is correctly aligned and the nervous system is functioning properly. To achieve this, the practitioner uses his or her hands or an adjusting tool to perform specific manipulations of the vertebrae. When these bones of the spine are not correctly articulated, resulting in a condition known as subluxation, the theory is that nerve transmission is disrupted and causes pain in the back, as well as other areas of the body.

Chiropractic is one of the most popular alternative therapies currently available. Some would say it now qualifies as mainstream treatment as opposed to complementary medicine. Chiropractic treatment is covered by many insurance plans and in 2004, the U.S. Department of Veterans Affairs announced full inclusion of chiropractic care for veterans. It has become well-accepted treatment for acute pain and problems of the spine, including lower back pain and whiplash...."

I didn't see anything in my research to connect this type of medicine and the kidneys, so I tried thinking about it another way. What are the major causes of Chronic Kidney Disease? We know diabetes is the first and hypertension the second.

I took a look at NaturalNews.com (https://www.naturalnews.com/035546_chiropractic_blood_sugar_diabetes.html) and found the following:

"The average person may not recognize how diabetes and chiropractic are connected. What does the back have to do with blood sugar? Often, an electrician understands this faster than most people. Interfere with the current flowing through the wires and the appliances or areas of the house lose normal function or might even catch fire.

If the nerve supply from the upper neck or middle back (the two areas that supply the pancreas) are disturbed, pancreatic function suffers; maybe in its ability to produce enzymes to digest proteins, fats and carbohydrates, or maybe insulin production, or both. Blood sugar and digestion become unbalanced, resulting in either in diabetes or hypoglycemia".

Nutritionist Carolyn Heintz further explains:

"Chiropractic care might be helpful to diabetics if problems in the spine affect blood flow to the pancreas. The pancreas releases insulin in the body which is necessary to regulate proper levels of glucose in the blood. If the pancreas is not receiving enough oxygen and nutrients through proper blood circulation, perhaps this might have an effect on insulin production.

Another way chiropractic treatment might help those who suffer from diabetes is by alleviating pressed nerves on the spine to allow for a regenerated connection between the brain and the systems that are involved in the endocrine system and a body's metabolism. Also, when the nervous system is free to work properly, the body can work to heal itself better."

You can read the rest of her article at http://belviderechiropractic.com/conditions/can-chiropractic-care-help-treat-diabetes/.

This makes sense. If there's a 'short' in the system, it's just not going to work. If you correct the short allowing the current to flow, you could be shortcutting diabetes... and maybe Chronic Kidney Disease.

Well, how about hypertension? How can chiropractic help with that?

This caught my eye, but it will need some explaining. I discovered it at https://www.echiropractor.org/chiropractic-blood-pressure/.

"Upper cervical chiropractic treatment, 'performed by a mechanical chiropractic adjusting device' was noted to decrease both systolic and diastolic blood pressures, and these findings were published in 1988.... More recently, it was found that the Atlas Adjustment lowered blood pressure with the effectiveness of 'two blood pressure medications given in combination', according to Dr. George Bakris. The drop in blood pressure as a result of the realignment of the Atlas vertebra was 'an average of 14 mm Hg greater drop' (systolic) and 'an average 8 mm Hg greater drop' (diastolic), compared to 'sham-treated patients'."

Cervical means

"relating or belonging to the neck, or to any body part that resembles a neck,"

according to Encarta Dictionary. In the paragraph above, it means the neck. A mechanical chiropractic adjusting device is used if more than finger or hand pressure is needed for spinal adjustment and sounds almost like a stapler. It doesn't break the skin, simply manipulates the spine.

The Atlas Adjustment is a little harder to explain. The topmost vertebra of your neck is called the Atlas because it holds up the globe better known as your head. Remember your Greek mythology? Atlas supported the world. It's this vertebra that is being manipulated.

I, for one, am convinced. I was wondering whether or not to continue the visits since I'm feeling better. It sounds like something I should do. How about you?

11/13/17 *Any Veterans Here?*

Veterans Day was Saturday, although many schools and business-
es chose to celebrate it on Friday. That confused me since I mis-
takenly thought all national holidays falling on the weekend in the
U.S. were celebrated on the following Monday. Once that was
straightened out for me, I wondered if we were the only country
to honor those who fought for us.

According to The United States Department of Veterans Affairs at
https://www.va.gov/opa/vetsday/vetday_faq.asp, we're not:

"Q. Is Veterans Day celebrated in other countries?

A. Yes, a number of countries honor their veterans each year on
November 11, although the name and types of commemorations
differ somewhat from Veterans Day celebrations in the United
States. For example, Canada and Australia observe 'Remembrance
Day' on November 11, and Great Britain observes 'Remembrance
Day' on the Sunday nearest to November 11. There are similarities
and differences between these countries' Remembrance Day and
America's Veterans Day. Canada's observance is actually quite similar to the U.S. celebration, in that the day is intended to honor all
who served in Canada's Armed Forces. However, unlike in the U.S.,
many Canadians wear red poppy flowers on November 11 in hon-
or of their war dead. In Australia, Remembrance Day is very much
like America's Memorial Day, a day to honor that nation's war
dead.

In Great Britain, the day is commemorated by church services and
parades of ex-service members in Whitehall, a wide ceremonial
avenue leading from London's Parliament Square to Trafalgar
Square. Wreaths of poppies are left at the Cenotaph, a war memorial in Whitehall, which was built after the First World War. At
the Cenotaph and elsewhere in the country, a two-minute silence

is observed at 11 a.m., to honor those who lost their lives in wars."

There are 600,000 veterans with kidney disease in the U.S. Considering that kidney disease is a medically dischargeable disease (Can you imagine soldiers in the field trying to stick to the renal diet?), I began to wonder just how our veterans were being treated once they were no longer active military.

I went to the National Institute of Diabetes and Digestive and Kidney Diseases at http://bit.ly/2ABGeli for the following information:

"The prevalence of chronic kidney disease (CKD) in the Veteran population is estimated to be 34% higher than in the general population, due to demographic differences and the existence of significant co-morbidities associated with CKD in the Veteran population—diabetes mellitus and hypertension. VA currently cares for over 600,000 Veterans with kidney disease in their 153 medical treatment facilities or 800 community based outreach clinics (CBOC's) across the United States. Those Veterans who progress to kidney failure are treated either at home or in one of the 70 VA dialysis units, or if dialysis services are not directly available, may be treated in the community under VA contracted care. Currently over 15,000 Veterans receive care directly by VA or through the community under VA contracted care. Eligible Veterans may also elect to receive dialysis care in the community using Medicare or other personal health benefits programs. Renal transplantation is also offered through the VA as a regionalized service at 5 centers."

Wait a minute. Why did "demographic differences and the existence of significant co-morbidities associated with CKD in the Veteran population—diabetes mellitus and hypertension" lead to a whopping 34% of veterans having kidney disease?

179

I know when Bear spoke with me about his 25 year military career, he talked of people with different ethnic backgrounds from different parts of the country... some from different parts of the world. I remembered writing this in *What Is It and How Did I Get It? Early Stage Chronic Kidney Disease*:

"...Native American, Alaskan Native, Hispanic, Pacific Islander or Afro-American ethnic groups...have a 15 to 17% higher occurrence of CKD."

And I was off and running. Last Veterans Day's Huffington Post was able to help out here.

"According to the U.S. Department of Defense, as of 2012 there were over 22,000 American Indians and Alaska Natives on active duty, and the 2010 Census identified over 150,000 American Indian and Alaska Native veterans."

You can read the entire article at https://www.huffingtonpost.com/national-museum-of-the-american-indian/american-indians-serve-in-the-us-military_b_7417854.html.

And Hispanics? Journalist Erika L. Sanchez wrote in 2013 that over 157, 000 Hispanics served in the military then. By the way, her article at http://nbclatino.com/2013/01/01/u-s-military-a-growing-latino-army/ gives the rest of us a little insight into the Latino community's military leanings.

I hesitate to come up with the number of Pacific Islanders serving in the military since the information is even older than that for Native Americans and Alaskan Natives (Did you notice they were grouped together?) or Hispanics. It's also included with that of Asians, so the categories are Asian-Pacific Islanders rather than Pacific Islanders.

As for Afro-Americans or Blacks – readers, which name do you prefer? – the closest I can figure out is that 370,842 Blacks or 16% of the Blacks in the United States served in the U.S. military... in 2011.

None of these statistics is current. It takes time for the military to collect and compose their data, but I had been hoping for numbers that were a little more timely.

And now the biggie: just how much is The Veterans Administration spending on veterans with kidney disease?

Finally, a fairly current article. In April of this year, MedPage Today at https://www.medpagetoday.com/meetingcoverage/nkf/64668 offered this information from Kristen Monaco's article:

"Rajiv Saran, MD, of the University of Michigan, and colleagues found the total cost of CKD care in the Department of Veterans Affairs healthcare system increased from $12 billion in 2006 to $19 billion in 2014 in current dollars. Adjusted for inflation, the increase was 26%, the researchers reported as a late-breaking abstract at the National Kidney Foundation's 2017 Spring Clinical Meeting.

More than three-fourths of the VA's aggregate spending each year on CKD patients was dedicated to patients with either stage 3a or 3b disease. However, the average cost per patient to treat increased with each worsening stage of CKD, with non-dialysis stage 5 CKD being the most expensive."

To all those who served, whether or not you developed kidney disease, thank you from the bottom of my heart.

11/20/17 *Giving Thanks*

Thursday is the American Thanksgiving. This is what we were taught in grade school when I was a child:

"In 1621, the Plymouth colonists and Wampanoag Indians shared an autumn harvest feast that is acknowledged today as one of the first Thanksgiving celebrations in the colonies. For more than two centuries, days of thanksgiving were celebrated by individual colonies and states. It wasn't until 1863, in the midst of the Civil War, that President Abraham Lincoln proclaimed a national Thanksgiving Day to be held each November."

Thank you History.com for that information.

Thanksgiving is celebrated in one form or another all over the world since it is basically a celebration of the harvest. For example, Canadians celebrate theirs on the second Monday of October since the harvest is earlier there. Then there's China's Mid-Autumn Moon Festival, Korea's Chuseok, the Liberian Thanksgiving, Ghana's Homowo Festival, and the Jewish Sukkot.

When Antidote, a clinical trial matching company I wrote about a few weeks ago asked me if I would be willing to be part of a video explaining what I thank medical research for, I jumped at the chance.

One thing all the different forms of Thanksgiving worldwide have is the delicious danger of overeating... and that is not good for our kidneys (no matter how scrumptious the food is). This report popped up on my news feed the other day. The source is Baylor College of Medicine.

"'The body absorbs nutrients from the gut and then the liver metabolizes them. Whatever is left that can't be used by the body is excreted by the kidneys,' said Mandayam, associate professor of medicine in the section of nephrology. 'The more you eat, the more you deliver to your kidneys to excrete, so eating a lot of substances that are very high in proteins or toxins can put a strain on your kidneys because they now have to handle the excess calories, toxins or proteins you've eaten.

During holidays like Thanksgiving, people tend to eat very heavy meals with lots of proteins and carbohydrates, and this can impact not only kidney function, but also liver, pancreas and cardiac function,' Mandayam said.

'When you consume carbohydrates, the body will use what is necessary for immediate energy release but any extra carbohydrates are converted into fat and stored underneath the skin and in the muscles and the liver. Similarly, when you eat a lot of fat, if the fat can't immediately be converted into energy-producing adenosine triphosphate, then all of the fat will be stored in various fat deposits in the body,' Mandayam explained.

'The building up of fat inside your liver can lead to liver failure or cirrhosis, and fat inside your blood vessels can lead to heart attacks. Additionally, eating a lot of protein that your body can't metabolize can lead to an increase in blood urea nitrogen, which adds stress on kidneys because they have to work harder to excrete this.

It is especially important for people with chronic kidney disease and kidney stones to not overeat,' he said.

'For people with kidney disease, even eating normal amounts of food puts stress on their kidneys,' he said. 'If you consume large amounts of carbohydrates, protein or fat the stress on an overworked, half functioning kidney will get even worse and can accelerate your kidney dysfunction.'"

It always made sense to me that overeating is detrimental to your health, but I was thinking in terms of obesity which could lead to diabetes which, in turn, could lead to CKD. I've also noticed that since I read this report, I've been eating less without making an effort. For years, I've been struggling with my weight and all I had to do is read this report????? Life is weird.

Let's talk about carbohydrates for a minute. I instantly think of bread, all kinds of bread which is even weirder because I've been on a low carb diet for a while. I know, you thought of cakes and pies, didn't you? Did you know that fruits and vegetables contain carbohydrates, too? That was a revelation to me.

Now I'm wondering about excess calories. I'm limited to 1200 a day and find that this is fine with me. Bear is larger, being both male and bigger than I am, so his calorie limitations are higher. Your renal dietician can tell you what your ideal calorie count per day is if you don't know.

So, why limit calories? Renal Medical Associates explain this succinctly:

"Why being overweight matters and what you can do about it.

We used to think that those 'few extra pounds' were just dead weight. We now know that those extra pounds work together to disrupt your body's normal functioning-with the goal of making you gain more weight. That's why losing weight is such a difficult task."

It's important to limit your calorie limit so that you don't add those extra pounds. The extra pounds not only make it more difficult to lose weight, but can lead to obesity... which can lead to diabetes... which can lead to CKD. This is starting to sound familiar, isn't it?

If you already have CKD, the extra pounds you gain without calorie restrictions make it more difficult for your poor, already over-worked and struggling kidneys to do their jobs.

What are those jobs you ask? Let's take a look at Verywell.com at https://www.verywell.com/kidney-functions-514154 's answer:

- **Prevent the Buildup of Waste Products** – The kidneys function as an intricate filter, removing normal waste products of metabolism, as well as toxins from the body. In the process of removing toxins, the kidneys may be damaged by these substances.
- **Regulate Fluid** – Through holding on to fluids when a person is dehydrated, or eliminating excess fluids, the kidneys control fluid balance in the body.
- **Regulate Electrolytes** – The kidneys play an important function in electrolyte balance in the body, regulating the levels of sodium, potassium, and phosphate. This maintaining of optimal levels of electrolytes is referred to as homeostasis - or equilibrium.
- **Regulate Blood Pressure** – Through the production of a hormone called renin, the kidneys play an important role in regulating blood pressure. Learn more about the renin-angiotensin system.
- **Regulate Production of Red Blood Cells** – The kidneys produce a hormone called erythropoietin which controls the production of red blood cells in the bone marrow.
- **Bone Health** - The kidneys produce an active form of vitamin D which keeps the bones healthy.

11/27/17 *Taming the Wild Weed*

I have a friend who is a kidney donor. That's actually how we met. I went to a conference to learn what I could learn and she was there at the invitation of the presenters. I was drawn to her right away not knowing who she was or why she was there... something about her magnetic personality, I think. That was years ago and since then I've attended her social media workshop and followed her closely on Instagram. Now she's involved with medical marijuana. That got me to thinking.

So I did a little searching. Back in 2013, the National Kidney Foundation answered a reader's question in their Ask the Doctor blog by responding more to the smoking than the marijuana:

"Smoking is not good for any person. Smoking is not safe for any person. I know of no specific ill effects of marijuana on the kidney."

It seemed to me something must have been discovered about medical marijuana and chronic kidney disease in the last four years, so I kept digging and found this 2014 article from Phoenix New Times at http://www.phoenixnewtimes.com/arts/can-i-get-a-medical-marijuana-card-for-chronic-kidney-disease-6577499:

"Medical-grade cannabis can help with pain management, but there are still alternating schools of thought as to whether weed helps or hurts the kidneys. Claims that marijuana injures the kidneys often point to smoking as a damaging factor, but there are alternative methods of ingesting cannabis, including vaporizing, tinctures, and infusing the drug into food.

Additionally, a joint study by the University of Calgary and the University of Alberta concluded that, 'Even small improvements in symptoms with the use of THC: CBD [cannabinoids, the active ingredients in cannabis] in patients with difficult-to-treat symptoms may be clinically meaningful.'

It seems, if you avoid smoking it, much more evidence exists that cannabis can help with the side effects of CRD, including nausea, loss of appetite, and weight loss."

CRD means Chronic Renal Disease, an alternative name for CKD. Well, that's a bit more informative, but still, three years old. By now I was curious to know how marijuana worked in the first place. United Patients Group at https://unitedpatientsgroup.com/resources/how-medical-marijuana-works had the answer and the date on their site was only last year.

"Major Cannabinoids in Medical Marijuana

What THC Is and Its Effects
THC stands for delta-9-tetrahydrocannibinol. It is probably the best known cannabinoid present in medical marijuana. Physically it acts as a muscle relaxant and anti-inflammatory and psychologically it acts as a stimulant. This makes medical marijuana strains high in THC a good choice for patients who need relief while also to remain alert and active.
THC in medical marijuana acts in the following ways:
- anti-epileptic
- anti-inflammatory
- anti-depressant
- stimulates appetite
- lowers blood pressure
- apoptosis (self induced cell death)

What CBD Is and Its Effects
CBD stands for cannabidiol. Cannabidiol actually reduces the psychological effects of medical marijuana. For most patients, a strain that has high THC and high cannabidiol will have fewer 'mental'

effects and more physical ones. High cannabidiol medical marijuana strains, like Blueberry and Harlequin, are especially effective for illnesses with strong physical symptoms. Cannabidiol's effects include:

- reduced pain
- reduced anxiety
- reduced nausea
- sedative effects
- anti-convulsive
- anti-schizophrenic
- arrests the spread of cancer

What CBN Is and Its Effects

CBN is cannabinol, not to be confused with Cannabidiol. Cannabinol is very similar to THC, but has less psychological effects. It is produced as THC breaks down within the medical marijuana plant. High THC will make cannabinol's effects stronger, and very high cannabinol concentrations can produce undesirably strong head highs. Cannabinol levels tend to be high in medical marijuana strains like Strawberry Haze and Blue Rhino, which can be particularly helpful for:

- lowering pressure in the eye (such as with glaucoma)
- analgesic
- anti-seizure

What CBC Is and Its Effects

CBC stands for cannabichromene. Cannabichromene's main action is to enhance the effects of THC. High cannabichromene levels will make a high-THC medical marijuana strain much more potent. Cannabichromene working together with THC is known to be a:

- sedative
- analgesic
- anti-inflammatory

What CBG Is and Its Effects

CBG is an abbreviation for cannabigerol. Cannabigerol has no psychological effects on its own, and is not usually found in high amounts in most medical marijuana. Scientists believe that cannabigerol is actually one of the oldest forms of cannabinoids, meaning it is essentially a 'parent' to the other cannabinoids found in medical marijuana. It also has anti-microbial properties. Cannabigerol has physical effects such as:

- lowering pressure in the eye
- anti-inflammatory
- sedative
- sleep assistance

Combining Strains

Alone, none of the five major cannabinoids are as effective as when they work together. These five cannabinoids also work with the minor compounds in marijuana, and this is probably one reason that medical marijuana replacements like Marinol do not work very well.

Professional medical marijuana growers can analyze their medical marijuana strains to breed and grow medication for patients with the desired range of levels of each major cannabinoid. Using this knowledge of what each compound does helps medical marijuana pharmacists, or budtenders, find the right combination for patients to treat specific conditions and find maximum relief."

I am not at a point where I would consider medical marijuana since my only symptoms are occasional brain fog and tiredness. Should I be experiencing the kind of pain some CKD users do, I would revisit this decision but I'd have to keep in mind that using this substance could hurt my chances of a transplant.

According to Joshua L. Rein, DO and Christina M. Wyatt, MD of the Division of Nephrology, Department of Medicine, Icahn School of Medicine at Mount Sinai, New York, NY as stated in their research study at http://www.ajkd.org/article/S0272-6386(17)30810-7/fulltext, as of this year:

"Twenty-nine US states have established medical marijuana programs, 8 of which have also legalized recreational marijuana, and Canada is expected to legalize recreational marijuana in 2018. Advanced chronic kidney disease (CKD) and end-stage renal disease (ESRD) are chronic conditions with significant associated morbidity and mortality."

Don't get confused. Medical marijuana is not a cure for CKD and is not suggested as one. However, should you have need of pain relief, it may offer you some… IF you live in a place where it is legal and IF your doctor thinks it's a good option for you.

12/4/17 *Movin' On Up*

Considering my family's history, I'm vigilant about having colonoscopies. This year, however, there was an additional test - an endoscopy. You may have heard of this as an upper endoscopy, EGD or esophagogastroduodenoscopy. The names are interchangeable. Whatever you call it, I was intrigued.

What is an endoscopy, you ask. According to the Mayo Clinic at https://www.mayoclinic.org/tests-procedures/endoscopy/basics/why-its-done/PRC-20020363:

"An upper endoscopy is used to diagnose and, sometimes, treat conditions that affect the upper part of your digestive system, including the esophagus, stomach and beginning of the small intestine (duodenum)."

Okay, but that doesn't explain what the procedure is. The National Institute of Diabetes and Digestive and Kidney Diseases at https://www.niddk.nih.gov/health-information/diagnostic-tests/upper-gi-endoscopy can help us out here:

"Upper GI endoscopy is a procedure in which a doctor uses an endoscope—a flexible tube with a camera—to see the lining of your upper GI tract. A gastroenterologist, surgeon, or other trained health care professional performs the procedure, most often while you receive light sedation to help you relax."

Relax? I was out like a light. First I was being shown was the device that was going to hold my mouth open and hold the tube that would be going down my throat, the next second I awoke in my room... or so it seemed.

Now the biggie: why have an endoscopy in the first place? I went to Patient Platform Limited at https://patient.info/health/gastroscopy-endoscopy and found this:

"A gastroscopy may be advised if you have symptoms such as:
- Repeated (recurring) indigestion.
- Recurring heartburn.
- Pains in the upper tummy (abdomen).
- Repeatedly being sick (vomiting).
- Difficulty swallowing.
- Other symptoms thought to be coming from the upper gut.

The sort of conditions which can be confirmed (or ruled out) include:
- Inflammation of the gullet (oesophagus), called oesophagitis. The operator will see areas of redness on the lining of the oesophagus.
- Stomach and duodenal ulcers. An ulcer looks like a small, red crater on the inside lining of the stomach or on the first part of the gut (small intestine) known as the duodenum.
- Inflammation of the duodenum (duodenitis) and inflammation of the stomach (gastritis).
- Stomach and oesophageal cancer.
- Various other rare conditions."

Wait a minute. I can already hear you asking what that has to do with Chronic Kidney Disease.

Claire J. Grant, from the Lilibeth Caberto Kidney Clinical Research Unit in London, Canada, and her colleagues' answer was reported in PhysciansEndoscopy at http://www.endocenters.com/chronic-kidney-disease-adversely-affects-digestive-function/#.WiLwjrpFxaQ,

"'CKD adversely affects digestive function,' the authors write. 'Abnormalities in digestive secretion and absorption may potentially have a broad impact in the prevention and treatment of both CKD and its complications.'"

Not good. We know that CKD requires close monitoring and life style changes. This may be another facet of the disease to which we need to pay attention.

I had some biopsies while I was under sedation. Nope, didn't feel a thing. But I now know I have gastritis and an irregular Z-line. The silver lining here is that I don't have Helicobacter pylori or H. pylori, a type of bacteria that infects the stomach which can be caused by chronic gastritis. Mine seems to be the food caused kind. Generally it's alcohol or caffeine, spicy foods, chocolate, or high fat foods that can cause this problem. I don't drink, eat spicy or high fat foods, and rarely eat chocolate, but noooooooooooooooooo, please don't take away those two luscious cups of coffee a day.

I wasn't sure what this Z-line thing was so started poking around on the internet, since I didn't catch it before seeing the gastroenterologist for my after visit appointment. Dr. Sidney Vinson, University of Arkansas for Medical Sciences/UAMS College of Medicine explained:

"This refers to the appearance of the tissue where the esophagus and stomach meet. The z-line is a zig-zag line where these 2 different type tissues meet. Occasionally it can be irregular and protrude more into the esophagus and not have the typical appearance. This is generally a benign condition but can occasionally represent mild barrett's esophagus, a precancerous change caused by reflux."

Apparently my normal duodenum was biopsied to see if my doctor could find a reason for the pain I was experiencing in the upper stomach. Well, it was more discomfort than pain, but he wanted to be certain there wasn't an ulcer... and there were no ulcers. Yay!

Hmmm, I have gastritis which is an inflammation and CKD, which is an inflammatory disease. Which came first? Did it matter? If I treat one will the other improve? I've been following the renal diet for all nine years since my diagnose and have made the appropriate life style changes, too.

What more could I do? There's the ever present to struggle to lose weight. That could help. I wasn't willing to take more medication as my gastroenterologist understood and accepted. I was already taking probiotics. I examined the little booklet produced by Patient Point that I was given more closely ignoring all the advertisements for medication.

Look at that. It seems sleeping on your left side can help. "Since your stomach curves to your left, part of it will be lower than your esophagus." I can do that, although I wonder if it will be awkward while wearing the BiPap.

I also learned that skipping late night snacks and eating smaller meals would be helpful since there would be less acid produced by smaller meals and I wouldn't have to deal with acid if I stopped eating at least two hours before bedtime. Acid is produced to help digest your food.

12/11/17 *Decisions, Decisions*

A reader asked me how I choose the articles or studies I include in the blogs. Now you've got to remember that researching and I go way back. I was fortunate in that Research Writing was my favorite course to teach before I retired as a community college instructor. I loved it.

I was going to give you my take on researching when I stumbled across Dr. Alicia White's piece on the United Kingdom's National Health Services site at https://www.nhs.uk/news/Pages/Howtoreadarticlesabouthealthandhealthcare.aspx. She's already written what I would have, so I'm dedicating today's blog to that. I have not reproduced all of it only because I don't have the room in the blog for that. Oh, those are not typos; they're the UK spelling. Take it away, Dr. White:

"If you've just read a health-related headline that has caused you to spit out your morning coffee ('Coffee causes cancer' usually does the trick), it's always best to follow the Blitz slogan: 'Keep Calm and Carry On'. On reading further, you'll often find the head-line has left out something important, such as: 'Injecting five rats with really highly concentrated coffee solution caused some changes in cells that might lead to tumours eventually (study funded by The Association of Tea Marketing).'

The most important rule to remember is: don't automatically be-lieve the headline. ..., you need to analyse the article to see what it says about the research it is reporting on....

Does the article support its claims with scientific research?
Your first concern should be the research behind the news article. If an article touts a treatment or some aspect of your lifestyle that is supposed to prevent or cause a disease, but doesn't give any information about the scientific research behind it, then treat it

with a lot of caution. The same applies to research that has yet to be published.

Is the article based on a conference abstract?
Another area for caution is if the news article is based on a conference abstract. Research presented at conferences is often at a preliminary stage and usually hasn't been scrutinised by experts in the field. Also, conference abstracts rarely provide full details about methods, making it difficult to judge how well the research was conducted. ...

Was the research in humans?
Quite often, the 'miracle cure' in the headline turns out to have only been tested on cells in the laboratory or on animals. ... Studies in cells and animals are crucial first steps and should not be undervalued. However, many drugs that show promising results in cells in laboratories don't work in animals, and many drugs that show promising results in animals don't work in humans. If you read a headline about a drug or food 'curing' rats, there is a chance it might cure humans in the future, but unfortunately a larger chance that it won't.....

How many people did the research study include?
In general, the larger a study the more you can trust its results. Small studies may miss important differences because they lack statistical 'power', and are also more susceptible to finding things (including things that are wrong) purely by chance. ... When it comes to sample sizes, bigger is usually better. So when you see a study conducted in a handful of people, treat it with caution.

Did the study have a control group?
.... If the question being asked is about whether a treatment or exposure has an effect or not, then the study needs to have a control group. A control group allows the researchers to compare

what happens to people who have the treatment/exposure with what happens to people who don't. ...

Also, it's important that the control group is as similar to the treated/exposed group as possible. The best way to achieve this is to randomly assign some people to be in the treated/exposed group and some people to be in the control group. This is what happens in a randomised controlled trial (RCT) and is why RCTs are considered the 'gold standard' for testing the effects of treatments and exposures. ... Without either, retain some healthy scepticism.

Did the study actually assess what's in the headline? .... For example, you might read a headline that claims: 'Tomatoes reduce the risk of heart attacks.' What you need to look for is evidence that the study actually looked at heart attacks. You might instead see that the study found that tomatoes reduce blood pressure. This means that someone has extrapolated that tomatoes must also have some impact on heart attacks, as high blood pressure is a risk factor for heart attacks. Sometimes these extrapolations will prove to be true, but other times they won't. Therefore if a news story is focusing on a health outcome that was not examined by the research, treat it with a pinch of salt.

Who paid for and conducted the study?
This is a somewhat cynical point, but one that's worth making. The majority of trials today are funded by manufacturers of the product being tested – be it a drug, vitamin cream or foodstuff. This means they have a vested interest in the results of the trial, which can potentially affect what the researchers find and report in all sorts of conscious and unconscious ways. This is not to say that all manufacturer-sponsored trials are unreliable. Many are very good. However, it's worth seeing who funded the study to sniff out a potential conflict of interest....."

Many thanks to Dr. White for her explanations.

Here we are in the middle of madness, holiday madness that is. Of course, that means we need to remind ourselves to slow down and destress. Exercising is one way to destress. We all have different ways to do that. The important thing is to do it... and stick to your renal diet if you follow one.

12/18/17 *Chemo and Kidneys*

Cancer has become an everyday word around here. While I have no personal acquaintance with cancer, too many friends and readers do. That got me to thinking. If you had chronic kidney disease and cancer, how would your already poorly functioning kidneys react to the chemotherapy?

We do need to start with some basics here. First, what is chemotherapy? According to the American Cancer Society at https://www.cancer.org/treatment/treatments-and-side-effects/treatment-types/chemotherapy/how-chemotherapy-drugs-work.html:

"More than 100 chemotherapy or chemo drugs are used to treat cancer – either alone or in combination with other drugs or treatments. These drugs are very different in their chemical composition, how they are taken, their usefulness in treating specific forms of cancer, and their side effects.

Chemotherapy works with the cell cycle
Chemotherapy drugs target cells at different phases of the process of forming new cells, called the cell cycle. Understanding how these drugs work helps doctors predict which drugs are likely to work well together. Doctors can also plan how often doses of each drug should be given based on the timing of the cell phases.

Cancer cells tend to form new cells more quickly than normal cells and this makes them a better target for chemotherapy drugs. However, chemo drugs can't tell the difference between healthy cells and cancer cells. This means normal cells are damaged along with the cancer cells, and this causes side effects. Each time chemo is given, it means trying to find a balance between killing the cancer cells (in order to cure or control the disease) and sparing the normal cells (to lessen side effects)."

Uh-oh, "normal cells are damaged along with the cancer cells." Let's see if we can get a bit more specific here and find out what happens to kidney cells. The Canadian Cancer Society at http://www.cancer.ca/en/cancer-information/diagnosis-and-treatment/chemotherapy-and-other-drug-therapies/chemotherapy/side-effects-of-chemotherapy/kidney-damage-and-chemotherapy/?region=on#ixzz51dnKcgtl offers the following information:

"Some chemotherapy drugs can damage the kidneys (nephrotoxicity). The kidneys break down and remove many chemotherapy drugs from the body. When chemotherapy drugs break down, they make products that can damage cells in the kidneys, ureters and bladder. The potential for kidney damage varies with the type of chemotherapy drug used.

Causes

Chemotherapy drugs that can cause kidney damage include:
- cisplatin (Platinol AQ)
- carboplatin (Paraplatin)
- nitrosureas, such as carmustine (BiCNU, BCNU)
- mitomycin (Mutamycin)
- methotrexate – especially if high doses are used
-
Whether or not a chemotherapy drug will cause kidney damage depends on:
- the dose of the drug used
- if other drugs, which also have the potential to damage the kidney, are used at the same time
- if the person already has kidney disease"

Look at the last item on the list. That's us; we already have kidney disease. Cancer.Net at https://www.cancer.net/navigating-cancer-care/older-adults/when-cancer-not-your-only-health-concern gives us just a bit more information about chemotherapy when you already have CKD. They also mention diabetes which is one of the leading causes of CKD.

"Diabetes. If you have diabetes, you need to monitor your blood glucose (blood sugar) levels closely during cancer treatment. Some chemotherapy and medications used to lower side effects (such as steroids) can raise your blood sugar levels. These levels might also go up because you are less physically active or under stress. Side effects like nausea and vomiting also affect your blood sugar.

Your doctor might also recommend:
- Taking low-sugar food supplements
- Taking different anti-nausea medications
- Using fast-acting insulin at times during cancer treatment
- Keeping a record of your blood sugar levels. You and your doctor can look at them during clinic visits. Controlling your blood sugar will help make sure you can stay on your cancer treatment schedule.

Kidney disease. Your kidneys might not work as well as you get older. So adults over 65 might have more problems with some types of chemotherapy. The drugs can be difficult for your kidneys to handle. This can raise your risk of kidney problems. How well your kidneys work might determine the type of chemotherapy you can have, or how often you have it.

If you are on dialysis, talk with your oncologist. Dialysis cleans your blood when your kidneys do not work well enough to do it. But dialysis may also clean the chemotherapy drugs out of your body before they can work."

This does address older adults which is why I believe they mention age as a CKD risk factor.

But there is hope. Take a look at what appeared in NDT (the *respected European Nephrology, Dialysis, Transplantation Journal*). It's a bit a technical, but you can read more of the study at https://academic.oup.com/ndt/article/30/12/1979/2459906:

"One of the important drug-related problems in patients with renal impairment is inappropriate medication use and dosing errors [105, 106]. Along this line, many cytotoxic drugs and their active/toxic metabolites are eliminated through the kidney depending on how much of the substance undergoes renal filtration, tubular secretion and/or tubular reabsorption. Hence, patients with both acute kidney injury (AKI) and CKD receiving chemotherapeutic agents often possess alterations in their pharmacokinetic parameters such as drug absorption, distribution, protein binding, biotransformation and renal excretion, which may result in the accumulation of potentially toxic components and over-dosage ....

Therefore, clinicians must be wary to appropriately adjust doses of drugs that are excreted primarily by the kidneys. This requires dosing according to the calculated or measured creatinine clearance or eGFR formulas, which will allow the safe use of chemotherapy in patients with underlying kidney disease."

Interesting to me is readers and friends' reactions to chemo. Some have none, other than high energy for a day or two after their treatment. Others are nauseous and depleted of energy. It depends on your unique body chemistry and the ingredients in your chemo cocktail (for lack of a better word).

Brag time! After being included in Healthline's Top Six Kidney Disease Blogs two years in a row, this year **SlowItDownCKD** has been awarded a place on BlogFeedSpot's Top 75 Nephrology Blogs GLOBALLY. You know that expression the British readers use – gob smacked? That's me!

12/25/17 *To Eat It or Not To Eat It*

Merry Christmas... and for tomorrow, Happy Kwaanza. Oh, all right, let's throw in Happy Chanukah although that's already passed this year. What all these celebrations – yes, and New Year's Eve, too – have in common is food. And food has potassium and phosphorous in it. Those are two of the electrolytes that Chronic Kidney Disease patients have to curtail.

Let's backtrack a little bit and find out what these are. Each was included in the glossary of *What Is It and How Did I Get It? Early Stage Chronic Kidney Disease*:

"Phosphorus: One of the electrolytes, works with calcium for bone formation, but too much can cause calcification where you don't want it: joints, eyes, skin, and heart.

Potassium: One of the electrolytes, important because it counter-acts sodium's effect on blood pressure."

Now, let's see if we can get a bit more information about the ill effects of having too much of either one. This is from *SlowItDownCKD 2011*:

"Be aware that kidney disease can cause excessive phosphorus. And what does that mean for Early Stage CKD patients? Not much if the phosphorous levels are kept low. Later, at Stages 4 and 5, bone problems including pain and breakage may be endured since excess phosphorous means the body tries to maintain balance by using the calcium that should be going to the bones."

And potassium? *SlowItDownCKD 2012* has the answer:

"Too much potassium can cause irregular heart beat and even heart attack. This can be the most immediate danger of not limiting your potassium."

We all have limitations on these (as well as sodium and protein) based upon our latest blood and urine lab results. Since my lab results registered normal for both electrolytes, I have pretty generous daily limitations: potassium: 3000 mg; phosphorous: 800 mg. If you're like me, the numbers didn't mean much.

Let's try this another way. My husband's traditional family Christmas dinner consists of standing rib roast, sweet potatoes baked in orange juice with marshmallow topping, string bean casserole, dinner rolls, tea or coke, and apple pie. (I added salad so there would be something I could eat.)

We'll need a list of high potassium and high phosphorous foods before we can to analyze the meal. Luckily, there is one for phosphorus in *SlowItDownCKD 2015*:

HIGH PHOSPHORUS FOOD TO LIMIT OR AVOID
Beverages:

ale	beer
chocolate drinks	cocoa
drinks made with milk	dark colas
canned iced teas	

Dairy Products:

cheese	cottage cheese
custard	ice cream
milk	pudding
cream soups	yogurt

Protein:

carp	crayfish
beef liver	chicken liver

fish roe

oysters

Vegetables:

dried beans and peas

black beans

garbanzo beans

lentils lima

pork'nbeans

soy beans

Other foods:

bran cereals

caramels

seeds

whole grain products

organ meats

sardines

baked beans

chick peas

kidney beans

northern beans

split peas

brewer's yeast

nuts

wheat germ

Now we need a list of high potassium foods. The National Kidney Foundation at https://www.kidney.org/atoz/content/potassium was helpful here. They also have a list for "Other Foods": Fruits and Vegetables:

Apricot, raw (2 medium) dried (5 halves)

Avocado (¼ whole)

Banana (½ whole)

Cantaloupe

Dates (5 whole)

Dried fruits

Figs, dried

boiled

Grapefruit Juice

Honeydew

Kiwi (1 medium)

Mango(1 medium)

Nectarine(1 medium)

Orange(1 medium)

Orange Juice

Acorn Squash

Artichoke

Bamboo Shoots

Baked Beans

Butternut Squash

Refried Beans

Beets, fresh then

Black Beans

Broccoli, cooked

Brussels Sprouts

Chinese Cabbage

Carrots, raw

Dried Beans and Peas

Greens, except Kale

Papaya (½ whole)
Pomegranate (1 whole)
Pomegranate Juice
Prunes
Prune Juice
cooked (½ cup)
Raisins
Parsnips
sweet
Pumpkin
Spinach, cooked
products
Vegetable Juices

Hubbard Squash
Kohlrabi
Lentils
Legumes
White Mushrooms,

Okra
Potatoes, white and

Rutabagas
Tomatoes/Tomato

Okay, here comes the hard part. Let's scan the lists to see which of the foods in the dinner my husband craved are on this list. I see canned iced teas, dark colas, orange juice, and sweet potatoes. The potassium and phosphorous in one serving (?) of each is as follows:

food	potassium	phosphorous
canned iced tea	18 mg.	32 mg.
dark cola	44 mg.	62 mg.
orange juice	235 mg.	40 mg.
sweet potatoes	542 mg.	81 mg.
totals	839 mg.	215 mg.

Doesn't look bad at all, does it? But it's all guesswork. Is your liquid serving an ounce? Eight ounces? What about the juice in the sweet potato dish? Surely it's not just one ounce. And maybe not eight depending upon how much of the juice is in the size portion of the sweet potato dish you had. Maybe you had seconds. Same for the sweet potatoes.

Since this is not at all a precise science, you're better off practicing more limiting rather than less. I'm not a doctor as I keep mentioning, but I don't see anything wrong with a just a taste or a small serving of each.

Of course, I'm not a fan of soda or any canned drink, so I get a pass on that. If you're not sure how much of what you can eat on a daily basis, make an appointment with your renal dietician after the holidays and just enjoy today's Christmas meal.

Hey, that doesn't give you free reign to eat all those things expressly not on your renal diet. I know if I decide to eat some of the standing rib roast, I'm still limited to five ounces of protein a day… including the hardboiled egg I had for breakfast.

Lay.off.the.salt.shaker.too. Sodium is not your friend if you have CKD. Ask your host if he or she has Mrs. Dash's seasoning or garlic powder (NOT SALT) should you be asked if you'd like the salt. Oh, was the green bean casserole made with canned, creamy soup? That's going to up the salt content. Just another thing to be aware of when salivating at the sight of the scrumptious meal in front of you today.

I'd go really light on the hot chocolate, too, if you were planning on having some. The message here is to enjoy, but limit, those high phosphorous and potassium holiday foods you really crave.

Until next year,
Keep living your life!

Index

My Notes -

Gail Rae-Garwood

Have you read my other Chronic Kidney Disease books? Available on Amazon.com and B&N.com (print and digital) or walk into a B&N to order them.

What Is It and How Did I Get It?
Early Stage Chronic Kidney Disease
SlowItDownCKD 2011
SlowItDownCKD 2012
The Book of Blogs: Moderate Stage Chronic Kidney
Disease
SlowItDownCKD 2015
SlowItDownCKD 2016

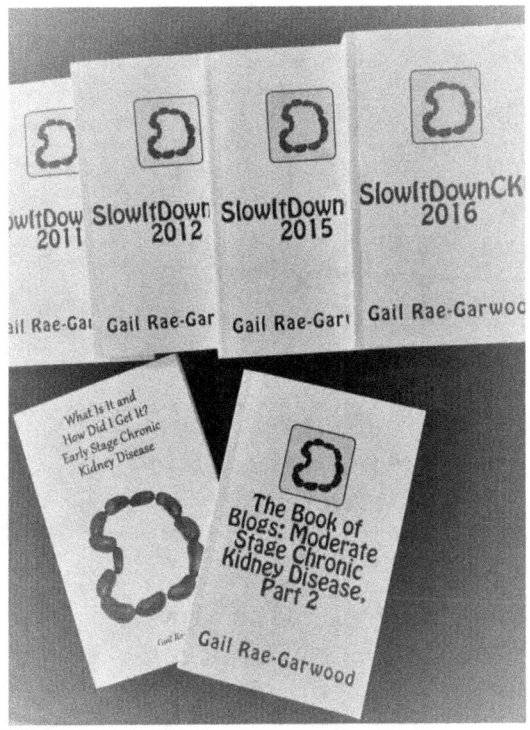

Follow the blog at
https://gailraegarwood.wordpress.com

SLOWITDOWNCKD
EARLY AND MODERATE STAGE CHRONIC KIDNEY DISEASE

On Instagram, Pinterest, and Twitter go to
@SlowItDownCKD

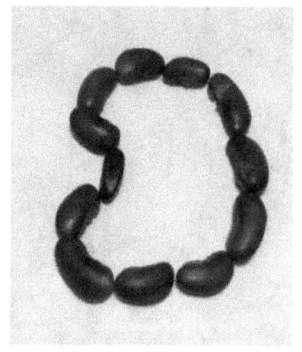

And then, there's the Facebook page at
*https://www.facebook.com/
SlowItDownCKD/*

Don't forget you can email me at
SlowItDownCKD@gmail.com

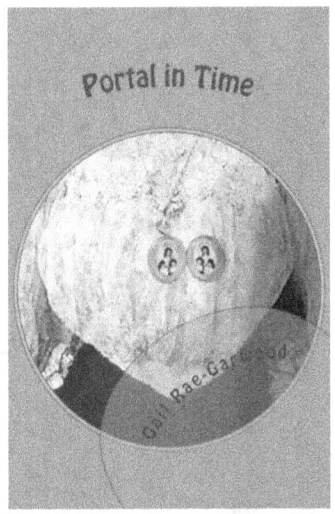

If you'd like to read a time travel romance (above) or fiction based on others' experiences (below), I've written one of each..

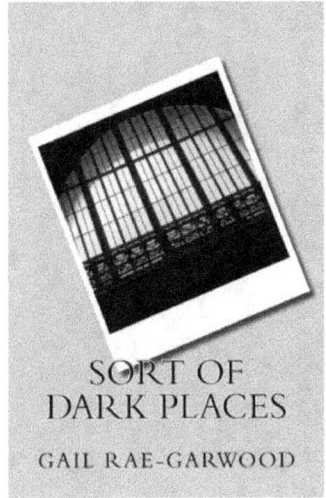

Gail Rae-Garwood